Sports-Related Injuries of the Meniscus

Guest Editor

PETER R. KURZWEIL, MD

CLINICS IN
SPORTS MEDICINE

www.sportsmed.theclinics.com

Consulting Editor
MARK D. MILLER, MD

January 2012 • Volume 31 • Number 1

SAUNDERS an imprint of ELSEVIER, Inc.

W.B. SAUNDERS COMPANY
A Division of Elsevier Inc.

1600 John F. Kennedy Blvd. • Suite 1800 • Philadelphia, Pennsylvania 19103

http://www.theclinics.com

CLINICS IN SPORTS MEDICINE Volume 31, Number 1
January 2012 ISSN 0278-5919, ISBN-13: 978-1-4557-3935-6

Editor: Jessica McCool

Clinics in Sports Medicine (ISSN 0278-5919) is published quarterly by Elsevier Inc., 360 Park Avenue South, New York, NY 10010-1710. Months of issue are January, April, July, and October. Business and Editorial Offices: 1600 John F. Kennedy Blvd., Ste. 1800, Philadelphia, PA 19103-2899. Customer Service Office: 3251 Riverport Lane, Maryland Heights, MO 63043. Periodicals postage paid at New York, NY and additional mailing offices. Subscription prices are $324.00 per year (US individuals), $503.00 per year (US institutions), $160.00 per year (US students), $367.00 per year (Canadian individuals), $608.00 per year (Canadian institutions), $223.00 per year (Canadian students), $446.00 per year (foreign individuals), $608.00 per year (foreign institutions), and $223.00 per year (foreign students). Foreign air speed delivery is included in all *Clinics* subscription prices. All prices are subject to change without notice. **POSTMASTER:** Send address changes to *Clinics in Sports Medicine,* Elsevier Health Sciences Division, Subscription Customer Service, 3251 Riverport Lane, Maryland Heights, MO 63043. Customer Service (orders, claims, online, change of address): Elsevier Health Sciences Division, Subscription Customer Service, 3251 Riverport Lane, Maryland Heights, MO 63043. Tel: 1-800-654-2452 (U.S. and Canada); 314-447-8871 (outside U.S. and Canada). Fax: 314-447-8029. E-mail: journalscustomerservice-usa@elsevier.com (for print support); journalsonlinesupport-usa@elsevier.com (for online support).

Reprints. For copies of 100 or more of articles in this publication, please contact the Commercial Reprints Department, Elsevier Inc., 360 Park Avenue South, New York, NY 10010-1710. Tel.: 212-633-3812; Fax: 212-462-1935; E-mail: reprints@elsevier.com.

Clinics in Sports Medicine is covered in *MEDLINE/PubMed (Index Medicus) Current Contents/Clinical Medicine, Excerpta Medica,* and *ISI/Biomed.*

Printed and bound by CPI Group (UK) Ltd, Croydon, CR0 4YY

Transferred to Digital Print 2012

Contributors

CONSULTING EDITOR

MARK D. MILLER, MD
S. Ward Casscells Professor of Orthopaedic Surgery, University of Virginia, Charlottesville, Virginia; Team Physician, James Madison University, Harrisonburg, Virginia

GUEST EDITOR

PETER R. KURZWEIL, MD
Southern California Center for Sports Medicine, Long Beach, California

AUTHORS

JIN HWAN AHN, MD
Professor in Orthopaedic Surgery, Sungkyunkwan University, School of Medicine, Kangbuk Samsung Hospital, Seoul, Korea

F. ALAN BARBER, MD, FACS
Plano Orthopedic Sports Medicine and Spine Center, Plano, Texas

SUE D. BARBER-WESTIN, BS
Cincinnati Sportsmedicine Research and Education Foundation, Cincinnati, Ohio

ANTHONY M. BARCIA, MD
Resident Physician, Orthopedic Surgery, Tripler Army Medical Center, Honolulu, Hawaii

ERIC D. BAVA, MD
Plano Orthopedic Sports Medicine and Spine Center, Plano, Texas

CORDELIA W. CARTER, MD
Clinical Fellow, Division of Sports Medicine, Children's Hospital Boston, Boston, Massachusetts

THOMAS M. DEBERARDINO, MD
Associate Professor, Department of Orthopaedics, University of Connecticut, Farmington, Connecticut

PETER D. FABRICANT, MD
Sports Medicine and Shoulder Department of Orthopaedic Surgery, Hospital for Special Surgery, New York, New York

DON JOHNSON, MD, FRCSC
Carleton University Sports Medicine Clinic, Ottawa, Ontario, Canada

MININDER S. KOCHER, MD, MPH
Associate Director, Division of Sports Medicine, Children's Hospital Boston; Associate Professor of Orthopaedic Surgery, Harvard Medical School, Boston, Massachusetts

ERICK J. KOZLOWSKI, BS, ATC
Certified Athletic Trainer, United States Air Force Academy, U.S. Air Force Academy, Colorado

SANG HAK LEE, MD
Assistant Professor in Orthopaedic Surgery, Kyung Hee University, School of Medicine, Kyung Hee University Hospital at Gangdong, Seoul, Korea

TRAVIS G. MAAK, MD
Sports Medicine and Shoulder Department of Orthopaedic Surgery, Hospital for Special Surgery, New York, New York

JOHN M. MARZO, MD
Associate Clinical Professor, Department of Orthopaedic Surgery, State University of New York, University at Buffalo, Buffalo, New York

GEORGIOS MOUZOPOULOS, MD, MSc
Center for Knee and Foot Surgery, Sports Traumatology, ATOS Clinic Heidelberg, Heidelberg, Germany

FRANK R. NOYES, MD
Cincinnati Sportsmedicine Research and Education Foundation, Cincinnati, Ohio

LAURA E. SCORDINO, MD
Orthopaedic Resident, Department of Orthopaedics, University of Connecticut, Farmington, Connecticut

RAINER SIEBOLD, MD, Priv-Doz
Center for Knee and Foot Surgery, Sports Traumatology, ATOS Clinic Heidelberg, Heidelberg, Germany

JOHN M. TOKISH, MD, LT COL, USAF MC
Program Director, Orthopedic Surgery, Sports Medicine, Tripler Army Medical Center, Honolulu, Hawaii

TIMOTHY R. VINYARD, MD
Resident, Department of Orthopaedic Surgery and Rehabilitation, University of Iowa Hospitals and Clinics, Iowa City, Iowa

WILLIAM M. WEISS, MD, MSc
Division of Orthopaedic Surgery, The University of Ottawa and Ottawa Hospital, Ottawa, Ontario, Canada

THOMAS L. WICKIEWICZ, MD
Sports Medicine and Shoulder Department of Orthopaedic Surgery, Hospital for Special Surgery, New York, New York

BRIAN R. WOLF, MD, MS
Associate Professor and Sports Medicine Fellowship Director, Department of Orthopaedic Surgery and Rehabilitation, University of Iowa Hospitals and Clinics; Head Team Physician, University of Iowa Athletics, Iowa City, Iowa

JAE CHUL YOO, MD
Associate Professor in Orthopaedic Surgery, Sungkyunkwan University, School of Medicine, Samsung Medical Center, Seoul, Korea

Contents

or in combination with other techniques for meniscal allograft transplants or synthetic meniscal replacements. Reported healing rates have met or exceeded those of other techniques.

Surgical techniques for repair of meniscus tears have expanded over the past couple of decades. The recent emergence of meniscal repair devices has allowed for minimally invasive techniques that can be employed with ease by most surgeons. Numerous devices from a multitude of manufacturers have become available and have increased the surgeon's options considerably. These meniscus fixation device designs have evolved rapidly over the past several years, making it difficult to keep up with the latest technological advances.

The value of the menisci for normal function of the knee joint is well documented. Meniscectomy often results in noteworthy damage to the knee joint, including deterioration of articular cartilage surfaces and subchondral bone sclerosis. Early investigations of meniscus repair that focused on simple longitudinal tears located in the periphery or outer one-third region reported high success rates. More recently, studies have documented satisfactory outcome of repair of complex multiplanar tears that extend into the central third avascular region.

Treatment of meniscal tears has shifted toward preservation, with meniscal repair when possible. Since the 1980s, biologic enhancement of meniscal repair has been reported. Initially fibrin clot was used to augment meniscal repairs in avascular zones of injury. Recently, the use of platelet-rich plasma has been applied to meniscal repair, particularly in avascular zones of injury. Although initial animal and clinical studies have shown promising results with the use of platelet-rich plasma to enhance meniscal repair, larger-scale, randomized trials with longer-term follow-up are needed to support its use. This article discusses the use of biologic products to enhance meniscal repair.

Meniscal root radial tears and avulsions occur frequently enough that one should be familiar with them as a clinical entity and recognize the typical clinical symptoms, MRI, and arthroscopic findings. The consequence of loss of the posterior horn attachment of the meniscus, according to best evidence, is loss of hoop strain constraint, meniscus extrusion, increased joint pressure, and premature degenerative disease of the knee over time. Surgical repair techniques are available, and the early-to-middle-range clinical results seem superior to those of nonoperative treatment or arthroscopic partial meniscectomy.

Meniscal repair represents the standard for treatment of vertical meniscal tears within the vascularized zone, if healing can be biologically expected. The development of all inside meniscus repair devices has been a turning point in the advancement of arthroscopic technique because of simplicity of implant insertion and the reduction in surgery time. The all-inside suture for peripheral longitudinal posterior horn tears using a posteromedial or posterolateral portal is an efficient and safe technique that provides anatomic coaptation of the torn meniscal fragment, an easy placement of vertically oriented suture, and a strong fixation, while minimizing the risk of neurovascular or chondral injuries.

Certain factors optimize the ability of meniscal tears to heal and these include younger age, acuity of injury, concomitant anterior cruciate ligament injury, simple tear type, smaller tear size, and peripheral location of tear (decreased rim width). Some types of meniscal tears are simply not amenable to surgical repair and, in these instances, judicious partial meniscectomy is indicated. Algorithms exist to help guide surgical decision-making, although definitive treatment for meniscal tears in the young patient should always be individualized, taking into account the patient's age, surgical history, concomitant injuries, and activity level.

Preservation of meniscal function is among the most important goals in knee surgery. Loss of this function after meniscal injury and treatment with meniscectomy has long been recognized to play a major role in the deterioration in knee function and the development of degenerative joint disease. Therefore, surgeons have become more and more aggressive with meniscal repair and adjunctive procedures to promote healing in meniscal surgery.

One method to repair symptomatic subtotal meniscus defect is to implant a meniscus scaffold at the site of the defect. Histology of preclinical and clinical biopsies of the implanted scaffold showed a repopulation of the scaffold by fibrous tissue and over time a remodeling of this fibrous tissue into fibrocartilaginous meniscuslike tissue. Although many clinical reports mentioned improvement in outcome scores, the clinical mid- to long-term efficacy of these implants on the prevention of osteoarthritis progression remains unclear, especially because there are no prospective, randomized, long-term studies comparing patients treated with meniscus scaffold implantation and control groups receiving only meniscectomy.

VISIT THE CLINICS ONLINE!

Access your subscription at:
www.theclinics.com

Foreword
Meniscal Repair

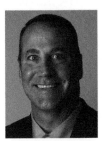

Mark D. Miller, MD
Consulting Editor

Although partial meniscectomy is perhaps the most common surgery done in orthopedics, meniscal preservation should always be our first thought. With this in mind, I invited one of the leaders in this area, Dr Peter Kurzweil from the Southern California Center for Sports Medicine, to assemble a team of experts to discuss this topic. The issue begins, like all surgical topics should, with indications. The standard meniscal repair options—inside-out, outside-in, and all-inside techniques are then discussed in detail. Extending indications and biologic enhancement of repair are topics that encourage us to "think outside the box" and try to repair more tears. Next, two contributions regarding posterior horn and root tears, a popular new topic, are covered. Pediatric meniscal tears is an important topic that has also been included. This is followed by recommendations for return to sport following repair. Finally, newer techniques for partial substitution in conjunction with meniscal excision are a new concept in meniscal preservation. One theme rings true throughout this issue—Save The Meniscus!

Mark D. Miller, MD
S. Ward Casscells Professor of Orthopaedic Surgery
University of Virginia
Team Physician, James Madison University
400 Ray C. Hunt Drive, Suite 330
Charlottesville, VA 22908-0159, USA

E-mail address:
mdm3p@virginia.edu

doi:10.1016/j.csm.2011.09.005

Preface

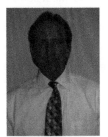

Peter R. Kurzweil, MD
Guest Editor

The evaluation and management of meniscus tears continues to be an evolving and dynamic segment of the sports medicine world. The goal of this issue of *Clinics in Sports Medicine* is to keep the interested practitioner up to date on the latest procedures and technologies involving the repair of meniscus tears.

This issue is written by a distinguished group of Sports Medicine specialists with expertise in various aspects of meniscus repair. The first article reviews indications for meniscus repair and the importance of meniscal preservation. The tried and true classic techniques of inside-out and outside-in suturing are updated while offering several surgical pearls. Meniscus Fixators continue to evolve and the latest generation of devices is discussed.

The next few articles concern particular meniscus tear patterns that were previously routinely treated with meniscectomy, but recently the trend has been to repair. This includes tears in the posterior root as well as tears in the avascular region. Biologic enhancement of the repair site is allowing the usual indications for what is considered to be a repairable tear to be stretched. Posterior horn tears are covered in a separate article demonstrating an all-inside suture repair without fixators. The repair of the posterior root is similar to anchoring a soft-tissue meniscal allograft posteriorly.

Speaking of allografts, this issue does not cover allografts, as that is a topic for a completely separate edition. Allografts generally require the complete removal of any remaining meniscal tissue prior to its replacement. Rather than sacrificing normal tissue, a new technology is currently being used by our European colleagues in which a scaffold is sutured into the meniscal defect to replace just the lost portion. This procedure is more equivalent to repairing a bucket handle tear rather than the larger operation required for an allograft. An article is devoted to this new technology and includes a discussion of the 2-year follow-up data. Although these meniscal scaffolds are not currently approved by the FDA, new trials are imminently forthcoming.

Meniscus tears in children also present a special circumstance as the knees can be smaller than adults. In addition, children have more years of heavy use of their knees ahead of them, all making the need for repair more vital. Hence, a separate article is devoted to this situation.

Clin Sports Med 31 (2012) xiii–xiv
doi:10.1016/j.csm.2011.09.011
0278-5919/12/$ – see front matter © 2012 Elsevier Inc. All rights reserved.

sportsmed.theclinics.com

Once meniscus repairs are complete, patients need to be guided back as they progressively increase their activity in preparation for returning to sports. Most current guidelines are based on assumptions regarding weight-bearing, strengthening, and presumed milestones. This issue will hopefully change many preconceptions and provoke changes in your current postoperative aftercare.

Peter R. Kurzweil, MD
Southern California Center for Sports Medicine
2760 Atlantic Avenue
Long Beach, CA 90806, USA

E-mail address:
pkurzweil@aol.com

Indications for Meniscus Repair

Travis G. Maak, MD*, Peter D. Fabricant, MD,
Thomas L. Wickiewicz, MD

KEYWORDS

- Meniscal tear • Knee injury • Meniscectomy
- Osteoarthritis • Meniscal repair

One of the earliest descriptions of the menisci was recorded by Bland-Sutton in 1897.[1] At that time, the menisci were thought to be vestigial tissue and were depicted as "the functionless remnants of intra-articular leg muscles."[1] Further advances in our understanding of the menisci have demonstrated that the menisci provide mechanical support and secondary stabilization, localized pressure distribution and load sharing, and lubrication and proprioception to the knee joint.[2,3]

When the menisci are injured, treatment is centered on both symptomatic relief (eg, pain and mechanical symptoms) as well as prevention of future sequelae (eg, osteoarthritis and cartilage degeneration). Many variables are considered in developing an operative treatment strategy after conservative management has failed. Patient-centered factors such as age, activity level, and physical fitness are important, as are characteristics of the meniscal tear itself such as size, location, and chronicity.

This review describes the function, anatomy, and biology of the menisci, discusses common mechanisms of injury and diagnostic strategies for localizing meniscal symptomatology, and highlights variables that are associated with improved prognosis for meniscal repair. Surgical indications for both meniscal tissue excision and salvage will be discussed, and an in-depth review of meniscal repair options will be presented.

FUNCTION AND ANATOMY OF THE MENISCUS

Both the macro- and microscopic anatomy of the menisci determines its function. The medial and lateral menisci are 2 C-shaped fibrocartilaginous structures attached anteriorly and posteriorly to the tibial plateau. The medial meniscus is longer in the anterior-posterior direction than the lateral meniscus and is continuous with the deep fibers of the medial collateral ligament and medial joint capsule, rendering it less

The authors have nothing to disclose.
The Sports Medicine and Shoulder Department of Orthopaedic Surgery, Hospital for Special Surgery, 535 East 70th Street, New York, NY 10021, USA
* Corresponding author.
E-mail address: maakt@hss.edu

Clin Sports Med 31 (2012) 1–14
doi:10.1016/j.csm.2011.08.012
0278-5919/12/$ – see front matter © 2012 Elsevier Inc. All rights reserved.

mobile. They function to provide mechanical support and secondary stabilization, localized pressure distribution and load sharing, and lubrication and proprioception to the knee joint.[2,3] The role of the meniscus as a secondary stabilizer of the knee is significant and has been quantified by Bedi and colleagues.[4] This study noted that transection of the anterior cruciate ligament (ACL) and meniscectomy resulted in nearly double the anterior tibial translation in both Lachman and pivot shift testing compared with that of the ACL alone, as measured with knee-specific computer navigation software. Mechanically, the menisci also transmit at least 50% to 75% of the axial load in knee extension and up to 85% with the knee in 90° of flexion.[5] When meniscal tissue is removed, as is the case with partial or total meniscectomy, the contact area of the knee joint (in both the same and opposite compartments) decreases, thereby increasing localized pressure on the surface of the articular cartilage. Increased pressure on the articular surface causes local cartilage damage, which leads to accelerated subchondral sclerosis and osteoarthritis.[6]

By dry weight, the menisci are comprised of mostly type I collagen (60%–70%), with a small amount of elastin (<1%) and other proteins (8%–13%).[7] Histologically, dense fibrocartilage is comprised of collagen fibers that are arranged circumferentially (to disperse compressive loads) with some radial fibers as well (to resist longitudinal tearing). At the surface, collagen fibers are arranged randomly to disperse shear stress associated with flexion and extension of the knee joint.[2] Proteoglycan macromolecules serve to hold and retain water, which is paramount to the compressive, shock-absorbing properties of the menisci and augments its ability to aid in lubrication of the knee joint. Finally, fibrochondrocytes exist sparsely dispersed throughout the meniscal tissue and act to synthesize extracellular matrix and support the acellular components of the menisci.

The blood supply of the menisci originates at the periphery in the perimeniscal capillary plexus, which are tributaries of the medial and lateral geniculate arteries. Importantly, only the peripheral 25% to 30% of meniscus is vascularized[8] (**Fig. 1**). The gradient attenuation in vascularity from the periphery to the central portion of the menisci is gradual but for ease of clinical classification led to the designation of 3 vascular "zones." The outer third is known as the *red-red zone* because of its relatively high concentration of vascular channels. In this zone, bleeding at the site if injury promotes fibrovascular scar formation and migration of anabolic cells in response to cytokines released during the inflammatory response. Because of this, tears in this zone have the highest healing potential. The middle vascular zone is termed the *red-white zone*. In this zone, there is intermediate vascularity, which leads to a less predictable result with regard to healing meniscal tears. If a repair is attempted in this zone, synovial abrasion, vascular access channels, and fibrin clot may be used to increase local blood flow and maximize healing potential. The red-red and red-white zones combine to form the outer 4 mm of the meniscus.[9] The remainder of the meniscus is avascular in adults and is therefore called the *white-white zone*. Nutrition of this tissue is achieved solely from the synovial fluid via passive diffusion, which is aided by motion of the knee joint. Consequently, injury in white-white zone of the meniscus does not stimulate a healing response, and there is a poor prognosis for healing after attempted repair.

MECHANISM OF INJURY AND DIAGNOSIS

Meniscal tears can be either traumatic or degenerative. Degenerative tears have been closely associated with osteoarthritis. Acute tears are often related to trauma, most frequently as a result of a twisting motion. Patients may or may not be able to recall a single traumatic event. Pain is often localized to the joint line and is usually

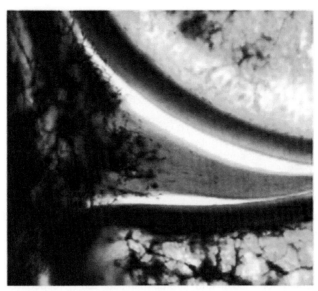

Fig. 1. Cross-sectional vasculature of the meniscus shows vascular supply to the peripheral 30% of the meniscus and the clear transition between red-red, red-white, and white-white zones.

intermittent. Constant pain or pain at rest usually indicates separate or additional pathology, such as osteoarthritis. Mechanical symptoms may also herald a meniscal tear, which include catching, locking, popping, pinching, or the feeling of having to move the knee through a specific range of motion to "reset" the joint. Effusion may or may not occur, and is not specific for meniscal pathology.

Physical examination typically finds joint line tenderness on the side of the meniscal tear. Pain with deep knee flexion is common for posterior horn injuries. Displaced tears may present with a mechanical block to range of motion that is also associated with distinct pain at that endpoint. Provocative maneuvers have been described that cause meniscal fragment impingement between the femoral and tibial surfaces. The McMurray test is performed on the medial meniscus by flexing the knee, creating a varus stress internally rotating the tibia, and bringing the knee into full extension. Reproducible pain with a palpable mechanical click or pop indicates a positive finding on the examination. Conversely, the lateral meniscus is tested with an applied valgus stress and external tibial rotation. Another commonly performed test is the Apley grind test, in which an axial load is created with concurrent internal and external rotation ("grind") with the patient positioned prone and the affected knee flexed to 90°. A positive examination is defined as pain at the medial or lateral joint line. A new clinical test, termed the *Thessaly test*, has been used to increase the diagnostic accuracy of the physical examination for meniscal tears by dynamically reproducing the load transmission in the knee joint at 5° and 20° of knee flexion. The Thessaly test is performed with the examiner holding the patient's outstretched hands while he or she performs a single leg stance flatfooted on the affected extremity and axially rotates 3 times with the knee in 5° and then 20° of flexion. A positive test result is documented with the presence of medial or lateral joint-line pain and possible mechanical symptoms. When this test is performed in 20° of flexion, 94% and 96% accuracy have

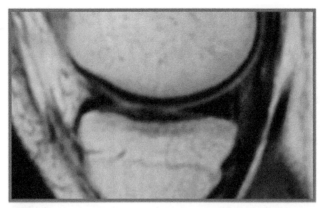

Fig. 2. Sagittal MRI shows a vertical tear through the vascular zone of the medial meniscus amenable to repair.

been documented for medial and lateral meniscal tears, respectively, with low false-positive and false-negative results.[10]

Plain x-rays should be the first-line radiographic study but are not sensitive or specific to meniscal pathology. Degenerative joint disease may indicate a degenerative meniscal tear, but acute tears have no specific radiographic findings. The ideal radiographic study to visualize meniscal pathology is magnetic resonance imaging (MRI; **Fig. 2**). It is important, however, to correlate MRI findings with the history and physical examination. Multiple studies have shown a high percentage of asymptomatic meniscal tears on MRI examination, ranging from 36%[11] to 76%.[12] This percentage increases significantly with patient age.[13] Prior MRI data from asymptomatic patients older than 65 years documented a 67% prevalence of meniscal tears.[14] This prevalence increased to 86% in the setting of symptomatic osteoarthritis.

RATIONALE FOR PRESERVATION OF MENISCAL TISSUE

Acute and chronic tears of the menisci are very common orthopedic injuries, affecting patients of various ages and activity levels. Meniscal injury often causes great pain and physical impairment, and clinical symptoms such as catching, locking, and decreased range of motion may frequently require surgical intervention for relief. The treatment for meniscal tears has adapted over the course of several decades with both technological and intellectual advances in orthopedic surgery. Since 1936, when total meniscectomy was the treatment of choice,[15] abundant research has led to the understanding that meniscal tissue should be retained whenever feasible.[16,17] For this reason, recent measures have attempted to preserve as much meniscus as possible. These measures have evolved from open total meniscectomy to open partial meniscectomy and finally to arthroscopic partial meniscectomy or repair. Meniscal injury was recently noted to be the most common musculoskeletal injury, occurring with a frequency of 23.8 per 100,000 per year.[18] Arthroscopic treatment of meniscal injuries has become one of the most common surgical procedures in the United States. The American Academy of Orthopedic Surgeons estimates that arthroscopy procedures of the knee total 636,000 cases per year in the United States as of 1999.[19] Within this cohort, arthroscopic treatment of meniscal injury is among the most common procedure performed, accounting for 10% to 20% of all surgeries at some centers.[20]

Long-term data are plentiful regarding the impact of surgical and demographic variables on the end result of removal of meniscal tissue.[21] A great deal of data have supported the hypothesis that increased meniscal resection predicts worse radiographic and functional long-term status.[22–26] Obesity[27,28] and advanced age[29,30] have been shown to be further predictive of even poorer functional and clinical result after resection of meniscal tissue. Data regarding medial versus lateral arthroscopic partial meniscectomy are mixed; although in vitro computer modeling postulates that lateral partial meniscectomy may lead to more degenerative changes when compared with medial partial meniscectomy,[31] in vivo studies have found no significant clinical differences.[29] Short- and medium-term analyses of outcomes regarding gender differences at 8.5 to 14.5 years after surgery show no difference in surgical outcome between men and women.[25,32,33] Nevertheless, 15- to 22-year follow-up data indicate that symptoms and functional limitations are worse in women who have undergone meniscectomy, compared with men,[30] and women tend to have more osteoarthritis.[27] Radiographic osteoarthritis is accelerated in patients with malalignment, as an even greater amount of stress is placed on the affected compartment.[32] Therefore, meniscal tissue is salvaged through meniscal repair whenever possible, and a substantial body of research has identified predictors of improved prognosis after meniscal repair.

SURGICAL INDICATIONS

The definitive treatment of meniscal tears involves either repair or excision of the pathologic tissue; however, not all patients with meniscal tears will require surgical intervention. Surgery is indicated in patients who have persistent mechanical symptoms and have not responded to a course of nonoperative treatment. Asymptomatic meniscal tears are common,[11–13] and the surgeon should be certain that a meniscal tear is the source of the patient's symptoms. The indications for arthroscopy include (1) symptoms of meniscal injury that affect activities of daily living, work, or sports, such as instability, locking, effusion, and pain; (2) positive physical findings of joint line tenderness, joint effusion, limitation of motion, and provocative signs, such as pain with squatting, a positive pinch test result, or a positive McMurray test result; (3) failure to respond to nonsurgical treatment, including activity modification, medication, and a rehabilitation program; and (4) ruling out of other causes of knee pain identified by patient history, physical examination, plain radiographs, or other imaging studies.[21,34]

After the decision has been made to proceed with arthroscopic intervention, an algorithm must be applied to guide specific treatment. The most important, and often most difficult, decision regarding treatment of meniscal tears is whether to excise or repair. Many factors must be considered during this decision-making process, including the tear location, tear type, tear etiology, concomitant injury, and patient profile. Consideration of each of these factors will optimize the final outcome after meniscal repair.

Tear Location

While every effort should be made to preserve meniscal tissue, several variables have been found to impact prognosis and healing rates after meniscal repair. As previously mentioned, tears in the vascular zones of the meniscus have the highest rates of healing.[35,36] Cannon and Vittori[35] reported a stepwise decline in healing rates as tear location moved from peripheral to central: 90% for tears within 2 mm of the periphery,

74% for tears within 3 mm of the periphery, and 50% for tears 4 to 5 mm away from the peripheral edge. It is this healing potential that restricts most repairs to within 4 to 5 mm from the peripheral edge. Nevertheless, repairs of tears with extension from the peripheral red-red or red-white zone into the central avascular zone have produced good outcomes, especially in the young, athletic population (see **Fig. 1**).[37]

In addition to the tear zone location, a tear located in the medial or lateral compartment may also impact healing potential. Prior data have documented improved healing in the lateral meniscus as compared with the medial meniscus.[35,38] However, other computed tomographic data from 53 patients failed to demonstrate a significant difference in healing between the 2 menisci.[39] Kalliakmanis and coworkers[40] also documented no difference in failure rates after medial and lateral meniscal repair for tears in the red-red and red-white zones in ACL-reconstructed knees. Although the impact of compartment on meniscal failure remains unclear, the poor outcomes after lateral meniscectomy have been well documented.[27] Therefore, the authors recommend applying a lower threshold for lateral meniscal repair.

Tear Type

Multiple types of tears have been described including vertical (longitudinal or circumferential), radial, horizontal (transverse or cleavage), degenerative, complex tear, and horn detachment; these types have been associated with variable healing potential. Multiple investigators have observed that tear type and configuration were predictive of outcome, with complex unstable tears (with greater than 3 mm displacement on examination with an arthroscopic probe) faring worse than simple vertical-longitudinal tear types.[36,41] Tear size was evaluated as well, and better results were seen after repair of tears longer than 8 to 10 mm.[36]

Recognition of the specific type of tear is crucial to guide treatment with meniscectomy or repair and to optimize healing after potential repair. Vertical tears are the most commonly repaired type of tear. This tear type is classically located less than 2 mm from the periphery and extends less than 2 cm in length (**Fig. 3**) Additionally, bucket-handle tears represent a subcategory of vertical tears that extend beyond 2 cm in length and have increased mobility.

Unlike vertical tears, radial tears are oriented perpendicular to the circumferential fibers and are commonly identified in the lateral meniscus after acute ACL rupture (**Fig. 4**). Again, variability exists in the length of these tears from small to large tears that extend from the white-white zone through to the periphery. A small radial tear involving less than 60% of the meniscus does not significantly influence compartment biomechanics, whereas a large radial tear that extends through greater than 90% of the meniscus to the periphery results in a significant increase in peak compartment pressures.[42] Therefore, radial tears should be stratified into partial (<90%) and complete (>90%) tears. Partial tears preserve the crucial peripheral circumferential fibers and thus the load distribution ability of the meniscus. This radial tear subtype can be debrided to a stable edge in most circumstances. Complete tears, however, result in complete circumferential fiber disruption, which not only compromises the function of the meniscus but also increases the biomechanical tendency for repair diastasis with axial load. Although diastasis significantly impairs healing, repair of this tear type should be attempted, as the only alternative treatment is an effective near-total meniscectomy. Particular care should be taken in the young patient given the importance of the meniscal load distribution in this population. Strict non–weight-bearing rehabilitation should be placed after repair of complete radial tears to reduce the potential for tear diastasis.

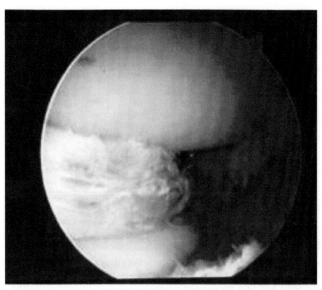

Fig. 3. Arthroscopic image shows a large vertical tear through the vascular meniscal zone. Note the reddish hue of the meniscus and capsule show the high vascular composition.

Horizontal tears often develop from variable shear stress between the superior and inferior meniscal regions in the early stage of meniscal degeneration. This tear type is commonly associated with meniscal cyst formation that may communicate with the periphery. These tears have been commonly identified on MRI; however, their

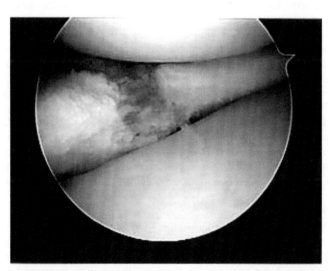

Fig. 4. Arthroscopic image shows a large radial tear extending to the periphery. Despite the decreased healing potential of this tear pattern, repair of the peripheral component should be attempted to minimize the complete destabilization of the meniscus. Strict non–weight bearing should be used postoperatively.

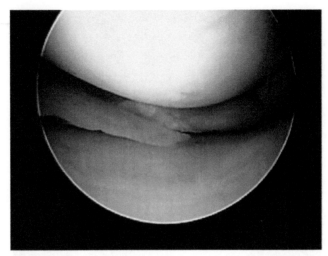

Fig. 5. Arthroscopic image shows a complex, degenerative type tear of the central avascular zone. Treatment of this tear type should include partial meniscectomy, as the healing potential of this zone and tear type is extremely low.

presence has not been linked to clinical symptoms.[43] Associated flap tears may be identified during diagnostic arthroscopy, yet the benefit of suture repair of these flaps remains unclear given the shear force orientation of the tear. Nevertheless, some data suggest that cyst aspiration and suture repair of the horizontal tear may obviate the need for meniscectomy.[44] In the opinion of the authors, most horizontal tears, including associated flaps, can be treated with partial meniscectomy.

Degenerative tears represent a continuation of the horizontal tear, typically in the aging population. Complex tears, including the parrot beak type and double longitudinal type, occur when the meniscal tissue is compromised in 2 or more planes and may represent a type of degenerative tear. This type of tear has a higher probability for failure, with particularly poor outcomes[45] documented with posterior segment tears compared with those extending into the middle segments (**Fig. 5**).[39] In most circumstances, these tear types can be either observed or excised if mechanical symptoms exist.

In addition to tear type, the length of the tear has been suggested to impact repair outcomes. This influence, however, remains unclear. Some data has suggested that an increased tear length may increase the risk and timing of repair failure. Cannon and Vittori[35] documented 90% and 50% healing rates with tears less than 2 cm and greater than 4 cm, respectively. Bach and colleagues[46] documented significantly earlier failure after repair in larger tears. Nevertheless, other data have been unable to document a significant difference in repair outcomes based on tear length.[9]

Tear Etiology

Acute tears have a higher rate of successful repair when compared with chronic ones; it is understood that repairs of tears less than 8 weeks old heal more frequently than older tears.[35] Additionally, patients undergoing repairs of traumatic meniscal tears have better 6-year functional results than do those with degenerative meniscal tears.[47,48] The majority of these studies, however, combine traumatic meniscal tear and concomitant injury. Stein and colleagues[49] recently compared long-term outcomes after arthroscopic meniscal repair versus partial meniscectomy for traumatic meniscal tears and documented no difference in function score. However, the meniscal repair group had a higher rate of return to preinjury and sporting activity levels. Additionally, only 40% of the meniscal repair group had osteoarthritic progression at 8-year follow-up as compared with 81% of the partial meniscectomy group. For these reasons, a recent traumatic history should be considered a good prognostic factor for meniscal healing within the meniscal repair algorithm.

Concomitant Injury

In addition to isolated meniscal pathology, concurrent structural knee injury can impact the success of meniscal repair. Long-term success of meniscal repair appears to depend on the stability of the knee at the time of surgery.[50] An increased probability for repairable tears exists in the setting of concomitant ligamentous injury. Meniscal repairs performed concurrently with ACL reconstruction have been reported to heal successfully upwards of 90% of the time, whereas repair without addressing knee stability often fails.[51] Review of published data in the ACL-deficient knee found a 92% overall success rate in meniscal healing after concurrent ACL reconstruction, whereas a 63% healing rate was documented without ACL reconstruction.[52] This increased healing rate is likely 2-fold—first, ACL reconstruction produces a hemarthrosis and fibrin clot that supplies intrarticular growth factors and a reparative scaffold for meniscal healing, and second, meniscal tears with concomitant ACL rupture are more commonly acute and traumatic, which has been associated with improved healing potential.[38,53] Prior outcome data obtained from a large multicenter study documented a 36% prevalence of combined ACL rupture and meniscal tear.[54] Longitudinal tears were most common and most frequently repaired, with other repaired types, including bucket-handle, complex, and horizontal. Nevertheless, the most frequent meniscal treatment procedure was partial meniscectomy. Therefore, although adherence to the indication criteria outlined in this article should be maintained, concomitant ACL rupture may allow an expanded threshold for meniscal repair.

Patient Profile

The influence of patient age on meniscal repair outcome has been well documented. Prior data have documented a reduced cellularity and healing response in patients older than 40 years.[55] Increased retear rates have also been documented in patients older than 30 years,[56] although failure occurred later in older patients.[46] The association between increased age and worse outcome seems to be negated in the setting of avascular tears and meniscal tears with concomitant ACL rupture. No difference between younger and older (40 to 58 years) patients has been found in clinical success after meniscal repairs performed in the avascular area.[45,57] Kalliakmanis and coworkers[40] recently documented no difference in repair failure between older or younger patients less than 35 years of age in the setting of concomitant ACL tear. Although prognostic factors, including avascular tears, concomitant ACL rupture, and continued ligamentous instability, seem to play identical roles in younger patients,[58] the consequence of postmeniscectomy arthritis remains significantly greater.

Synthesis

One may synthesize surgical indications for meniscal repair from the above variables that can predict healing prognosis. Contraindications for repair include older or sedentary patients or patients that are unable to perform the necessary postoperative rehabilitation. Additionally, isolated inner-third white-white tears with a remaining rim greater than 6 mm should not be repaired. Borderline tears, including middle-third white-white tears should only be considered for repair if extension exists into the red-white or red-red region. Degenerative or stable, longitudinal (<12 mm in length) tears should also not be repaired. Meniscal tears with a rim greater than 4 mm should be considered for repair, as removal of this large tear will result in biomechanics similar to a total meniscectomy.[59] Particular consideration should be given in this circumstance to patients younger than 40 years and those with active lifestyles. Meniscal repair is ideal in younger patients with acute, traumatic tears. Healing potential is maximized if tears are in the vascular red-red zone or are vertical-longitudinal tears greater than 12 mm. Varus or valgus malalignment is unfavorable for medial or lateral meniscal repair, respectively. Meniscal tissue should be fixed where appropriate during ACL reconstruction, with favorable results in both the red-red and red-white zones. Of course, patient compliance with postoperative rehabilitation protocols and weight-bearing restrictions is paramount to a successful repair, and inability to comply may be a contraindication for meniscal salvage procedures. Conversely, excision is therefore favored in older patients with degenerative, chronic tears, tears in the avascular white-white zone, and unstable tears.

COMPLICATIONS AND CONSIDERATIONS

Complications after meniscal repair include chondral injury, implant failure, postoperative joint-line irritation, nerve injury, arthrofibrosis, effusion, infection, deep venous thrombosis, and pulmonary embolus.[60,61] Bleeding or pseudoaneurisms may occur after meniscal surgery but are primarily associated with posterior horn resection and not meniscal repair.[62,63] Nerve injury has also been documented with meniscal repair techniques. Medial meniscal repair has been associated with injury to the saphenous nerve producing transient neuropraxia, but permanent injury has only been identified in 0.4% to 1% of documented cases.[64-66] Peroneal nerve injury is a rare but devastating injury that may occur during lateral meniscal repair. A carefully dissected posterolateral safety incision with proper retractor placement will significantly reduce this risk.[67] Retrospective, consecutive data documented a 20% and 14% complication risk with and without meniscal repair and concomitant ACL injury, respectively.[60] The most commonly encountered complications were saphenous neuropathy and arthrofibrosis. A 13% and 19% risk was documented for lateral and medial repairs, respectively. Additionally, a significantly higher complication rate was identified in female patients. Kurzweil and coworkers[61] documented similar findings, including the presence of a postoperative pulmonary embolus.

SUMMARY

The roles of the menisci in force transmission and chondral protection within the knee have been well documented. The range of repairable meniscal tears is expanding because of recent augmentation techniques and improved understanding of meniscal healing. Identification of repairable meniscal tears is crucial to healing success and improved outcomes. Careful consideration should be given to the factors that may contribute to or inhibit meniscal healing including tear location, tear type, tear etiology, concomitant injury, and patient profile. Treatment of all identified repairable meniscal tears should be managed carefully to maximize the healing potential after repair. Focus should be placed on optimizing the biological environment and mechanical stability of the repaired meniscus to maximize healing. Finally, the outcomes of meniscal repair should be reported to aid the current understanding of meniscal healing and improve this crucial process.

REFERENCES

1. Bland-Sutton J. Ligaments, their nature and morphology. Philadelphia: P. Blakiston; 1887.
2. Greis PE, Bardana DD, Holmstrom MC, et al. Meniscal injury: I. Basic science and evaluation. J Am Acad Orthop Surg 2002;10(3):168–76.
3. McDermott ID, Amis AA. The consequences of meniscectomy. J Bone Joint Surg Br 2006;88(12):1549–56.
4. Bedi A, Maak T, Musahl V, et al. Effect of tibial tunnel position on stability of the knee after anterior cruciate ligament reconstruction: is the tibial tunnel position most important? Am J Sports Med 2011;39(2):366–73.
5. Ahmed AM, Burke DL. In-vitro measurement of static pressure distribution in synovial joints—Part I: tibial surface of the knee. J Biomech Eng 1983;105(3):216–25.
6. Ihn JC, Kim SJ, Park IH. In vitro study of contact area and pressure distribution in the human knee after partial and total meniscectomy. Int Orthop 1993;17(4):214–8.
7. Bullough PG, Munuera L, Murphy J, et al. The strength of the menisci of the knee as it relates to their fine structure. J Bone Joint Surg Br 1970;52(3):564–7.
8. Arnoczky SP, Warren RF. Microvasculature of the human meniscus. Am J Sports Med 1982;10(2):90–5.
9. Kimura M, Shirakura K, Hasegawa A, et al. Second look arthroscopy after meniscal repair. Factors affecting the healing rate. Clin Orthop Relat Res 1995;(314):185–91.
10. Karachalios T, Hantes M, Zibis AH, et al. Diagnostic accuracy of a new clinical test (the Thessaly test) for early detection of meniscal tears. J Bone Joint Surg Am 2005;87(5): 955–62.
11. Zanetti M, Pfirrmann CW, Schmid MR, et al. Patients with suspected meniscal tears: prevalence of abnormalities seen on MRI of 100 symptomatic and 100 contralateral asymptomatic knees. AJR Am J Roentgenol 2003;181(3):635–41.
12. Bhattacharyya T, Gale D, Dewire P, et al. The clinical importance of meniscal tears demonstrated by magnetic resonance imaging in osteoarthritis of the knee. J Bone Joint Surg Am 2003;85-A(1):4–9.
13. Boden SD, Davis DO, Dina TS, et al. A prospective and blinded investigation of magnetic resonance imaging of the knee. Abnormal findings in asymptomatic subjects. Clin Orthop Relat Res 1992;(282):177–85.
14. Bhattacharyya T, Gale D, Dewire P, et al. The clinical importance of meniscal tears demonstrated by magnetic resonance imaging in osteoarthritis of the knee. J Bone Joint Surg Am 2003;85-A(1):4–9.
15. King D. The healing of semilunar cartilages. 1936. Clin Orthop Relat Res 1990;(252): 4–7.
16. McGinity JB, Geuss LF, Marvin RA. Partial or total meniscectomy: a comparative analysis. J Bone Joint Surg Am 1977;59(6):763–6.
17. Northmore-Ball MD, Dandy DJ, Jackson RW. Arthroscopic, open partial, and total meniscectomy. A comparative study. J Bone Joint Surg Br 1983;65(4):400–4.
18. Clayton RA, Court-Brown CM. The epidemiology of musculoskeletal tendinous and ligamentous injuries. Injury 2008;39(12):1338–44.
19. Praemer A, Furner S, Rice DP. Musculoskeletal conditions in the United States. Vol 2. Park Ridge (IL): American Academy of Orthopaedic Surgeons; 1999.
20. Renstrom P, Johnson RJ. Anatomy and biomechanics of the menisci. Clin Sports Med 1990;9(3):523–38.
21. Fabricant PD, Jokl P. Surgical outcomes after arthroscopic partial meniscectomy. J Am Acad Orthop Surg 2007;15(11):647–53.

22. Andersson-Molina H, Karlsson H, Rockborn P. Arthroscopic partial and total menis-cectomy: A long-term follow-up study with matched controls. Arthroscopy 2002; 18(2):183–9.
23. Bonneux I, Vandekerckhove B. Arthroscopic partial lateral meniscectomy long-term results in athletes. Acta Orthopaedica Belgica 2002;68(4):356–61.
24. Englund M, Roos EM, Lohmander LS. Impact of type of meniscal tear on radiographic and symptomatic knee osteoarthritis: a sixteen-year followup of meniscectomy with matched controls. Arthritis Rheum 2003;48(8):2178–87.
25. Higuchi H, Kimura M, Shirakura K, et al. Factors affecting long-term results after arthroscopic partial meniscectomy. Clin Orthop Relat Res 2000;(377):161–8.
26. Meredith DS, Losina E, Mahomed NN, et al. Factors predicting functional and radiographic outcomes after arthroscopic partial meniscectomy: a review of the literature. Arthroscopy 2005;21(2):211–23.
27. Englund M, Lohmander LS. Risk factors for symptomatic knee osteoarthritis fifteen to twenty-two years after meniscectomy. Arthritis Rheum 2004;50(9):2811–9.
28. Harrison MM, Morrell J, Hopman WM. Influence of obesity on outcome after knee arthroscopy. Arthroscopy 2004;20(7):691–5.
29. Chatain F, Adeleine P, Chambat P, et al. A comparative study of medial versus lateral arthroscopic partial meniscectomy on stable knees: 10-year minimum follow-up. Arthroscopy 2003;19(8):842–9.
30. Roos EM, Ostenberg A, Roos H, et al. Long-term outcome of meniscectomy: symptoms, function, and performance tests in patients with or without radio-graphic osteoarthritis compared to matched controls. Osteoarthritis Cartilage 2001;9(4):316–24.
31. Pena E, Calvo B, Martinez MA, et al. Why lateral meniscectomy is more dangerous than medial meniscectomy. A finite element study. J Orthop Res 2006;24(5): 1001–10.
32. Burks RT, Metcalf MH, Metcalf RW. Fifteen-year follow-up of arthroscopic partial meniscectomy. Arthroscopy 1997;13(6):673–9.
33. Fauno P, Nielsen AB. Arthroscopic partial meniscectomy: a long-term follow-up. Arthroscopy 1992;8(3):345–9.
34. Metcalf RW, Burks RT, Metcalf MS, et al. Arthroscopic meniscectomy. Operative arthroscopy, vol. 3. Philadelphia: Lippincott Williams & Wilkins; 1996. p. 263.
35. Cannon WD Jr, Vittori JM. The incidence of healing in arthroscopic meniscal repairs in anterior cruciate ligament-reconstructed knees versus stable knees. Am J Sports Med 1992;20(2):176–81.
36. DeHaven KE. Meniscus repair. Am J Sports Med 1999;27(2):242–50.
37. Noyes FR, Barber-Westin SD. Arthroscopic repair of meniscal tears extending into the avascular zone in patients younger than twenty years of age. Am J Sports Med 2002;30(4):589–600.
38. Morgan CD, Wojtys EM, Casscells CD, et al. Arthroscopic meniscal repair evaluated by second-look arthroscopy. Am J Sports Med 1991;19(6):632–7[discussion: 637–8].
39. Pujol N, Panarella L, Selmi TA, et al. Meniscal healing after meniscal repair: a CT arthrography assessment. Am J Sports Med 2008;36(8):1489–95.
40. Kalliakmanis A, Zourntos S, Bousgas D, et al. Comparison of arthroscopic meniscal repair results using 3 different meniscal repair devices in anterior cruciate ligament reconstruction patients. Arthroscopy 2008;24(7):810–6.
41. Hanks GA, Kalenak A. Arthroscopy update #7. Alternative arthroscopic techniques for meniscus repair. A review. Orthop Rev 1990;19(6):541–8.

42. Bedi A, Kelly NH, Baad M, et al. Dynamic contact mechanics of the medial meniscus as a function of radial tear, repair, and partial meniscectomy. J Bone Joint Surg Am 2010;92(6):1398–408.
43. Noble J. Lesions of the menisci. Autopsy incidence in adults less than fifty-five years old. J Bone Joint Surg Am 1977;59(4):480–3.
44. Lu KH. Arthroscopic meniscal repair and needle aspiration for meniscal tear with meniscal cyst. Arthroscopy 2006;22(12):1367,e1361–4.
45. Rubman MH, Noyes FR, Barber-Westin SD. Arthroscopic repair of meniscal tears that extend into the avascular zone. A review of 198 single and complex tears. Am J Sports Med 1998;26(1):87–95.
46. Bach BR Jr, Dennis M, Balin J, et al. Arthroscopic meniscal repair: analysis of treatment failures. J Knee Surg 2005;18(4):278–84.
47. Menetrey J, Siegrist O, Fritschy D. Medial meniscectomy in patients over the age of fifty: a six year follow-up study. Swiss Surg 2002;8(3):113–9.
48. Shelbourne KD, Carr DR. Meniscal repair compared with meniscectomy for bucket-handle medial meniscal tears in anterior cruciate ligament-reconstructed knees. Am J Sports Med 2003;31(5):718–23.
49. Stein T, Mehling AP, Welsch F, et al. Long-term outcome after arthroscopic meniscal repair versus arthroscopic partial meniscectomy for traumatic meniscal tears. Am J Sports Med 2010;38(8):1542–8.
50. Jager A, Starker M, Herresthal J. Can meniscus refixation prevent early development of arthrosis in the knee joint? Long-term results. Zentralblatt fur Chirurgie 2000;125(6):532–5.
51. Turman KA, Diduch DR. Meniscal repair: indications and techniques. J Knee Surg 2008;21(2):154–62.
52. Bellabarba C, Bush-Joseph CA, Bach BR Jr. Patterns of meniscal injury in the anterior cruciate-deficient knee: a review of the literature. Am J Orthop (Belle Mead NJ) 1997;26(1):18–23.
53. Arnoczky SP, Warren RF, Spivak JM. Meniscal repair using an exogenous fibrin clot. An experimental study in dogs J Bone Joint Surg Am 1988;70(8):1209–17.
54. Fetzer GB, Spindler KP, Amendola A, et al. Potential market for new meniscus repair strategies: evaluation of the MOON cohort. J Knee Surg 2009;22(3):180–6.
55. Mesiha M, Zurakowski D, Soriano J, et al. Pathologic characteristics of the torn human meniscus. Am J Sports Med 2007;35(1):103–12.
56. Eggli S, Wegmuller H, Kosina J, et al. Long-term results of arthroscopic meniscal repair. An analysis of isolated tears Am J Sports Med 1995;23(6):715–20.
57. Noyes FR, Barber-Westin SD. Arthroscopic repair of meniscus tears extending into the avascular zone with or without anterior cruciate ligament reconstruction in patients 40 years of age and older. Arthroscopy 2000;16(8):822–9.
58. Krych AJ, McIntosh AL, Voll AE, et al. Arthroscopic repair of isolated meniscal tears in patients 18 years and younger. Am J Sports Med 2008;36(7):1283–9.
59. Lee GP, Diduch DR. Deteriorating outcomes after meniscal repair using the Meniscus Arrow in knees undergoing concurrent anterior cruciate ligament reconstruction: increased failure rate with long-term follow-up. Am J Sports Med 2005;33(8):1138–41.
60. Austin KS, Sherman OH. Complications of arthroscopic meniscal repair. Am J Sports Med 1993;21(6):864–8[discussion: 868–9].
61. Kurzweil PR, Tifford CD, Ignacio EM. Unsatisfactory clinical results of meniscal repair using the meniscus arrow. Arthroscopy 2005;21(8):905.

62. Jeffries JT, Gainor BJ, Allen WC, et al. Injury to the popliteal artery as a complication of arthroscopic surgery. A report of two cases. J Bone Joint Surg Am 1987;69(5): 783–5.

63. Tawes RL Jr, Etheredge SN, Webb RL, et al. Popliteal artery injury complicating arthroscopic menisectomy. Am J Surg 1988;156(2):136–8.

64. Barber FA, Click SD. Meniscus repair rehabilitation with concurrent anterior cruciate reconstruction. Arthroscopy 1997;13(4):433–7.

65. Small NC. Complications in arthroscopic surgery performed by experienced arthroscopists. Arthroscopy 1988;4(3):215–21.

66. Small NC. Complications in arthroscopic meniscal surgery. Clin Sports Med 1990; 9(3):609–17.

67. Deutsch A, Wyzykowski RJ, Victoroff BN. Evaluation of the anatomy of the common peroneal nerve. Defining nerve-at-risk in arthroscopically assisted lateral meniscus repair. Am J Sports Med 1999;27(1):10–5.

Meniscal Repair Using the Inside-Out Suture Technique

Don Johnson, MD, FRCSC[a],*, William M. Weiss, MD, MSc[b]

KEYWORDS

• Meniscal repair • Inside-out technique • Arthroscopic surgery
• Complications • Post-operative management

Injuries to the knee menisci are common, with a reported annual incidence of 60 to 70 per 100,000.[1] Operations to treat meniscal injuries rank among the most frequent procedures performed by orthopedic surgeons, and it is estimated that in some centers 10% to 20% of all surgeries are for meniscal tears.[1] However, before addressing any meniscal pathology, a firm grasp of the basic science related to the gross and microscopic anatomy, blood supply, and regenerative capacity of the menisci is required. Ongoing research into the natural history, basic science, and biomechanics of meniscal injury has called attention to the importance of preserving the meniscus to protect the articular surfaces of the knee.[2]

Annandale[3] reported the first meniscal repair in 1885, contradicting conventional wisdom of the time characterizing menisci as functionless remnants of muscle origins.[4] Our understanding of meniscus function has since evolved to its current status as a crucial component of the normal biomechanics of the knee. The first arthroscopic meniscus repair was reported in 1979 by Ikeuchi,[5] which has since renewed interest in this procedure and the ability to perform it arthroscopically. Our growing understanding of meniscal function has revealed its importance in tibio-femoral load transmission, shock absorption, lubrication, and passive stabilization of the knee.[6–8] Removal of meniscal tissue is known to decrease the contact surface area within the knee, increasing stress on the articular cartilage proportional to the meniscus removed, inevitably resulting in radiographic changes and symptomatic degeneration the knee cartilage.[9–15] As evidence of the development of degenerative changes after meniscectomy accumulates, surgeons have become increasingly aggressive in their efforts to conserve the meniscus.[6]

The senior author is a consultant for Arthrex.
[a] Carleton University Sports Medicine Clinic, 1125 Colonel By Drive, Ottawa, ON K1S5B6, Canada
[b] Division of Orthopaedic Surgery, The University of Ottawa and Ottawa Hospital, General Campus, 501 Smyth Road, Ottawa, ON K1H 8L6, Canada
* Corresponding author.
E-mail address: johnson_don@rogers.com

Numerous meniscal repair techniques have been described, but there remains no consensus among experts as to which is most effective.[16] These have evolved from an open repair with sutures to arthroscopic techniques using diverse tools and implants. Many of these devices have facilitated meniscal repair, making it more appealing and accessible to the arthroscopic knee surgeon.

The arthroscopic inside-out suture repair originally described by Henning and Lynch[10] is currently the gold standard by which other techniques are judged, with reported success rates of up to 90%, although what makes the inside-out technique the gold standard are still only level IV studies. The zone-specific method popularized by Rosenberg uses a single-lumen cannula system (Linvatec, Largo, FL, USA) to reach all zones of the meniscus through which sutures for meniscus repair are passed.[17] Modifications of this technique have also been described, which include use of a malleable cannula and flexible Nitinol needles for suture passage (Arthrex, Naples, FL, USA).[18,19] The use of a double slotted cannula for suture passage has also been described, eliminating the need for repositioning but allowing only horizontal suture placement.[20] Devices such as the Sharp-Shooter Meniscal Repair System (Linvatec) allow the surgeon more control in suture placement using only one hand. However, biomechanical studies have found that the suture configuration is more important to stability of the repair than the system used, and the vertical loop configuration has been shown to be twice as strong as the horizontal.[21] Multiple vertical loops of nonabsorbable suture placed 5 mm apart on the superior and inferior surface provides the most stable repair and is the configuration used in this investigation.

INDICATIONS

Several tear characteristics must be considered before choosing to repair a meniscus, including the location, size, appearance, chronicity, and the presence of secondary tears. Patient factors, such as age, activity, compliance with rehabilitation, and anterior cruciate ligament (ACL) injury must also be taken into account. The decision to repair or resect the meniscus must be individualized for each tear and patient.

Meniscal tears less than 25 mm in length are more amenable to repair than those more extensive, and the ideal tear type for fixation is a vertical longitudinal split (**Fig. 1**). Peripheral meniscus tears have the greatest potential for healing and, therefore, repair, as this area represents the red-red and red-white zones named according to

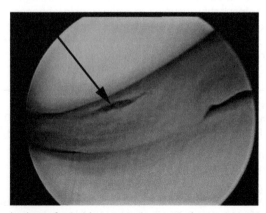

Fig. 1. An ideal meniscal tear for inside-out repair, a vertical posterior peripheral tear (*arrow*).

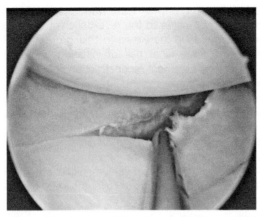

Fig. 2. The tear is probed with a hook to determine vascularity and stability.

their degree of vascularity (**Fig. 2**). Surgical repair of lateral meniscus tears have more favorable outcomes than those in the medial meniscus and thus have broader indications. Flaps, degenerative tears, and horizontal cleavage tears are not considered repairable (**Fig. 3**). In complex tears, all components are probed and assessed for their potential to heal. Rarely, all components of a complex tear are repairable. More commonly, a central bucket handle portion is excised and the peripheral aspects of the tear are repaired. No benefit has been observed from the repair of horizontal or radial tears, and tears of the central portion of the meniscus are best treated with debridement. Acute tears are more likely to heal with repair, whereas chronic tears are more often degenerative and better treated with meniscectomy. It is our opinion that chronic tears with no signs of delamination that remain anatomically reduced through knee flexion should be repaired.

Historically, partial meniscectomy has been recommended for patients older than 45 years with meniscal tears and stable knees, but acceptable results with repairs

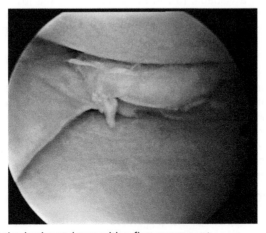

Fig. 3. A degenerative horizontal tear with a flap component.

have been reported in this age group for tears with appropriate characteristics.[22,23] Special consideration must be given to the ACL-deficient knee, as failure rates for meniscal repair are known to be increased in this group.[24] Without the stability provided by the ACL, the knee is at risk of initiating new meniscus tears and propagating preexisting ones. Ligament reconstruction should be considered for the ACL-deficient knee with a repairable meniscal tear.[24,25]

As a result of the biologic stimulation and stability conferred by the procedure, stable meniscal tears may be treated conservatively when identified at the time of ACL reconstruction. Stable tears include those that do not displace when probed, are less than 10 mm long, are in the posterior horn of the medial or lateral meniscus, and have been found to be asymptomatic despite conservative treatment[26,27] or after trephination.[28,29] However, stable longitudinal medial meniscal tears have been shown to have a higher propensity to propagate and fail over time and may be better managed with meniscal repair.[30]

The ideal candidate for meniscal repair is a young patient with a 2-cm vertical longitudinal tear in the peripheral 3 mm of the red-red or red-white zone and is undergoing concomitant ACL reconstruction.

PREOPERATIVE PLANNING

Meniscal tears commonly result from a twisting injury during sports participation, but they may also occur from age-related degeneration with no history of trauma. The acute injury is typically followed by recurrent episodes of pain localized to the joint line, and pain may be accompanied by swelling and mechanical symptoms, such as clicking or locking.

Tenderness to palpation along the joint line is among the most sensitive signs of meniscal tear, but joint effusion, quadriceps atrophy, or lack of full knee range of motion may also be noted on examination. Tests to assess meniscal integrity, such as the McMurray and Apley grind tests, may not be conclusive but can aid in diagnosis. The collateral and cruciate ligaments are assessed to determine the presence of additional injury. Finally, the knee is examined for signs of degenerative arthritis.

Radiologic evaluation of a suspected meniscal tear should include routine anteroposterior (AP) and lateral x-rays of the knee. If degenerative changes are expected, standing views including a 45° flexion AP view should be performed to assess joint space narrowing. Although not clinically indicated in all patients, magnetic resonance imaging (MRI) plays a valuable role in the evaluation of the full range of meniscal pathology. With more than 90% accuracy in determining the presence of a meniscal tear,[31,32] MRI has become widely accepted as an accurate noninvasive technique for its evaluation.[33]

Initial treatment of meniscal tears is based on patient symptoms. Conservative management may be successful in patients who have minimal pain and swelling and full range of motion and are willing to modify their activities. However, if symptoms persist, surgical intervention may be indicated. Patients who present with a locked knee, which lacks full extension, are likely to have a displaced bucket-handle tear requiring acute surgical intervention.

Although it is extremely difficult to identify meniscal tears amenable to repair preoperatively, a thorough patient assessment will aid the decision to repair or excise. The most important surgical principle is the preservation of functional meniscal tissue.

SURGICAL TECHNIQUE

Inside-out meniscus repair can be performed as outpatient surgery, using either general or regional anesthesia. Regardless of anesthesia type, patients also receive

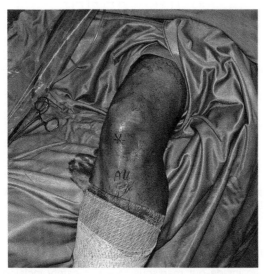

Fig. 4. The knee must be prepared and draped to allow circumferential access.

an injection of local anesthesia at the incision sites after the preparation and drape and before incisions are made.

Patient Position and Diagnostic Arthroscopy

The patient must be positioned to allow circumferential access to the affected knee and should be prepared and draped to allow posteromedial and posterolateral incisions should they be required (**Fig. 4**). This is accomplished by placing the patient supine, such that the break in the table is at the level of the tourniquet, which allows knee flexion to 90°. Alternatively, a leg holder can be used that allows abduction of the leg away from the operating table and then knee flexion as needed. Diagnostic arthroscopy is performed using a 30° arthroscope and includes an evaluation of both menisci, the articular cartilage of the knee, and the cruciate ligaments. The menisci are probed on the inferior and superior surfaces to identify tears. When assessing meniscal stability, it is important to note that the lateral meniscus is normally more mobile than the medial.[34] An unstable meniscus tear is defined as longer than half the length of the meniscus, which can be subluxed under the condyle when probed. Although a tourniquet may be used to improve visualization during the procedure, some surgeons prefer to leave it deflated for the diagnostic arthroscopy to assess the vascularity of the meniscal tear after rasping. The tourniquet should be placed on the proximal thigh at a minimum distance of 20 to 30 cm (10 to 12 inches) from the joint line.

Medial meniscus repairs are performed in some degree of knee extension (15° to 45° of flexion) depending on the location of the tear, to allow adequate visualization and access. Laterally, optimal visualization is obtained with the knee flexed and the leg in the figure-of-four position. This position also protects the peroneal nerve, which lies posterior to the biceps femoris tendon and furthest from the joint capsule with the knee in flexion.

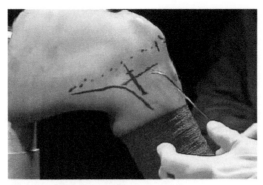

Fig. 5. The skin incision on the medial side of the knee is posterior to the medial collateral ligament and anterior to the saphenous nerve.

The Posteromedial and Posterolateral Incision

When performing an inside-out meniscus repair, a safety incision is made on the appropriate side of the knee with the joint in flexion. The incision should be just distal to the joint line, as sutures are passed in a cranio-caudal direction.

On the medial side, a 2- to 3-cm skin incision is made posterior to the medial collateral ligament and is carried through fascia along the anterior border of the sartorius muscle (**Fig. 5**). The sartorius is retracted posteriorly, protecting the saphenous vein and nerve lying deep to its posterior border. Care should be taken to protect the infrapatellar branch of the saphenous nerve, which penetrates the sartorius to become superficial to the fascia at the joint line. Using blunt dissection, the interval between the posteromedial capsule and the medial head of the gastrocnemius is opened, just proximal to the semimembranosus tendon.

On the lateral side, the joint line, lateral collateral ligament, and fibular head are identified before making an incision posterior to the lateral collateral ligament (**Fig. 6**). The incision is extended 3 cm distal to the joint line, with the knee at 90° of flexion. This approach is continued bluntly between the biceps femoris posteriorly and the iliotibial band anteriorly. The superior lateral geniculate vessels can be coagulated if encountered. The biceps femoris is retracted posteriorly, protecting the peroneal

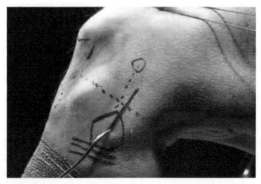

Fig. 6. The incision on the lateral side of the knee is posterior to the lateral collateral ligament at the level of the joint line.

nerve, which lies posterior and medial to the biceps tendon at this level. The lateral head of the gastrocnemius is identified, and dissection proceeds between the gastrocnemius and capsule where a retractor can be placed during the passage of sutures.

An alternate method of site selection for the safety incision is to pass the meniscal probe over the tear and apply an outward pressure from inside the knee. The probe can be palpated from the skin surface and then utilized for placement of the incision.

Preparing the Meniscus

After identification, the meniscal tear should be probed to determine its suitability for repair. Bucket-handle tears are typically reduced using the blunt arthroscope trochar before examination. The tear edges are debrided of degenerate fibrous tissue using a rasp or small shaver. Abrasion of the menisco-synovial junction is also performed, as it is believed to improve the success rate of repair independent of repair method.[35,36]

Zhang and coworkers[37] found that the meniscus may be trephinated to produce vascular access channels by removal of a core of tissue from the periphery of the meniscus, adjacent to the tear, connecting the avascular portion to the peripheral blood supply. This can be performed either with multiple passes of an 18-gauge needle from the outer surface of the knee through the meniscal tear or using one of the anterior portals through the meniscal tear into the peripheral rim and capsule (**Fig. 7**). Zhang and coworkers[37,38] continue to champion this technique and have shown increased healing rates and decreased symptoms when trephination is performed during repair.

Inside-Out Meniscal Repair Techniques

The major advantages of the inside-out meniscal repair technique are its versatility, ease of use, relatively short learning curve, and reliability. Excellent healing rates using

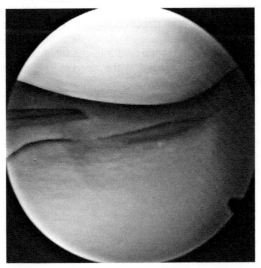

Fig. 7. Trephination with an 18-gauge spinal needle to puncture the periphery of the meniscus and produce vascular access channels.

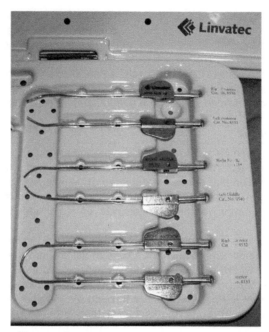

Fig. 8. The zone-specific cannula system.

this technique have been widely reported in the literature.[37,39–46] The zone-specific system popularized by Rosenberg and colleagues[18] in 1986 uses a single-lumen cannula system (Linvatec) through which sutures are passed (**Fig. 8**). The system includes 6 different curvatures of cannula, which allow the surgeon access to every part of the meniscus. They also have a 15° upward curve, which allows the cannula to be placed against the meniscus, the suture to be passed parallel to the joint line from a slightly elevated portal, access to the meniscus around obstacles like the tibial spines and femoral condyles, and direction of the needles away from posterior neurovascular structures. A malleable cannula system (Arthrex) is also helpful to manipulate the cannula over the spines and into a satisfactory position (**Fig. 9**). A posterior retractor is essential for retrieving the needles and to prevent inadvertent migration of the tips (**Fig. 10**).

Meniscal tears are routinely repaired using anterior portals, with the arthroscope in the ipsilateral portal and the cannula in the contralateral portal. The appropriate cannula is placed against the meniscus adjacent to the tear, and a 2-0 high-strength suture attached on both ends to 10-inch needles is then passed (**Fig. 11**). The high-strength suture is stronger than the 2-0 braided polyester that was previously used. It is very disconcerting to break the suture when tying it over the posterior capsule, and thus the extra strength is appreciated. Be careful that you do not pull the suture back and forth and have it cut through the meniscus. If the loop is slightly loose, I tie the front to the back suture on the outside to take out the slack. Before passing the suture, the needle can be passed through the central part of the meniscal tear, thus providing control of it for anatomic reduction (**Fig. 12**). A retractor is placed in the posterior safety incision to protect the neurovascular structures and can be used to deflect the needles into the wound, aiding the assistant who retrieves them (**Fig. 13**). After passage of the first needle through the wound, tension is applied to the

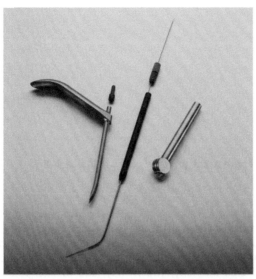

Fig. 9. The malleable cannula system, with a tip that can be directed to access difficult areas.

suture to prevent it from kinking and being cut within the cannula. The cannula is readjusted to enable placement of a vertical mattress suture, and the second needle is passed. This process is then repeated, placing stitches every 3 to 5 mm along the length of the tear (**Fig. 14**). Once all sutures are passed, the needles are removed, and the sutures are tightened and sequentially tied over the capsule. The probe is then used to verify the reduction and stable fixation of the meniscal tear.

Large bucket-handle tears that extend into the posterior aspect of the meniscus represent a unique situation. The posterior horn component of the tear is difficult to access and repair using the inside out technique, and the risk of injuring the posterior neurovascular bundle in doing so is high. Therefore, this type of tear is better addressed with a hybrid repair, which entails the use of an inside-out repair with

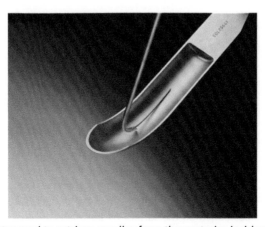

Fig. 10. The retractor used to retrieve needles from the posterior incision.

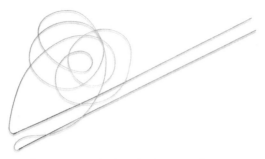

Fig. 11. The high-strength suture attached to the long needles.

vertical suture placement to reduce and fix the bucket-handle tear and an all-inside technique for the posterior horn component. It is often necessary to place a suture under the meniscus to adequately reduce and secure the torn fragment (**Fig. 15**). If this step is not completed, the meniscus may heal only on the superior surface and leave an unhealed cleft inferiorly, which may lead to later retear because of the incomplete healing. For tears in the anterior one-third of the meniscus, the preferred method is to use outside-in sutures.

RESULTS

The reported results of the inside-out meniscal repair technique in the literature have been excellent. Miller's[47] early study consisted of 87 patients with 116 meniscus tears, 96 of which were repaired. Only 19 patients (27%) had isolated meniscal injuries, and stabilizing procedures were performed on all patients with ACL-deficient knees. At follow-up, 79 repairs were assessed at a mean of 39 months (12 months–5.5 years), and a 91% success rate in retaining the meniscus was found. This investigation concluded that the time from injury to repair did not affect meniscal healing, but associated stabilization of ACL deficiencies is imperative for success.

Cannon and Vittori[48] found that lateral meniscal repairs fare better than medial, and a smaller rim width yields better overall healing. Patients with ACL reconstruction had

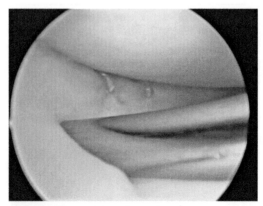

Fig. 12. The cannula positioned on the surface of the meniscus to pass the needles from inside to outside.

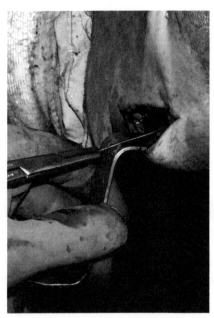

Fig. 13. Retrieving the needle deflected off the metal retractor in the posteromedial incision.

better results than those with isolated meniscal repair, regardless of tear length. Older patients had better healing than younger ones, and acute repairs were more successful than chronic.

Brown and colleagues[41] showed that 92% of meniscal tears with rims less than 4 mm were asymptomatic after repair, and the patients returned to sport.

Perdue and coworkers[39] examined 63 patients who underwent inside-out meniscus repair using a malleable cannula. After a mean follow-up of 27 months, 45 patients were available for clinical examination. Tegner and Lysholm scores were

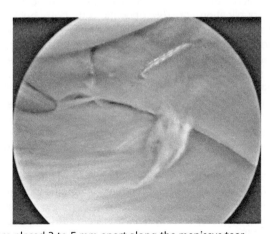

Fig. 14. Sutures are placed 3 to 5 mm apart along the meniscus tear.

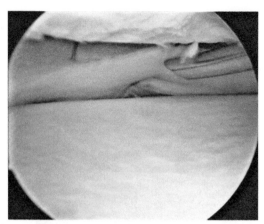

Fig. 15. In bucket-handle tears, the sutures should also be placed on the inferior surface.

64% excellent and 27% good, with outcomes independent of age, gender, and length of the meniscal tear.

Ryu and Dunbar[49] repaired 31 menisci, with the majority (29 of 31) being in the red-red or red-white zones and vertical bucket-handle tears of the posterior horn averaging 25 mm in length. Clinical healing was present in 27 of 31 (87%) repaired menisci.

Ventakatchalam and colleagues[50] retrospectively examined the outcomes of meniscal repairs in an attempt to identify factors that might improve results. In 60 meniscal repairs, the overall success rate was only 66.1%. Repair within 3 months of injury had a better prognosis than later repair. Healing rates of atraumatic meniscal tears were much lower than that for traumatic tears, 42% and 73%, respectively. An isolated atraumatic medial meniscus tear had particularly poor results, with only 33% healing, and may be more appropriate for meniscectomy.

Shelbourne and Rask[29] showed that repaired unstable peripheral vertical medial meniscus tears have a failure rate of 13.6%, with most recurrences occurring after more than 2 years. Of stable peripheral vertical medial meniscus tears treated with abrasion and trephination, most (94%) remained asymptomatic without stabilization. In a more recent publication, of 155 patients with both bucket-handle medial meniscus and anterior cruciate ligament tears, 56 menisci underwent repair and 99 that were deemed degenerative underwent meniscectomy.[51] After 6 to 8 years, functional outcomes showed that patients with repaired degenerative tears had significantly lower subjective scores than those with nondegenerative tears.

Hantes and colleagues[52] published a prospective, randomized, controlled trial comparing the inside-out zone-specific meniscal repair with outside-in and all-inside repairs. The study assessed 57 patients with longitudinal meniscal tears measuring more than 10 mm on preoperative MRI, with concomitant ACL tear present in 51%. At a mean follow-up of 22 months, the inside-out technique resulted in a higher success rate of meniscal repair with shorter operating times.

Choi and colleagues[53] compared all-inside repair of red-red zone tears with inside-out repair of red-white tears or red-red tears extending into the central zone, all in conjunction with ACL repair. Of the 14 patients undergoing all-inside repair and 34 with inside-out repair, meniscal healing rates were similar (71.4 and 70.6%, respectively) on follow-up MRI examination at a mean of 35.7 months.

Logan and coworkers followed up with 45 inside-out meniscal repairs in elite athletes, 83% of which also underwent ACL repair, for an average of 8.5 years. Failure, defined as symptoms of recurrent meniscal tear or repeat arthroscopy with meniscectomy, was seen in 26.7%. However, after eliminating failures because of repeat trauma, the failure rate was only 11%. In terms of performance, 81% of those with meniscal repair were able to return to their previous level of competition.

COMPLICATIONS

Although rare, complications can occur despite appropriate preventive measures. In a prospective 19-month study of complications experienced by arthroscopists, Small[54,55] reported a complication rate of 1.29%. Potential risks of arthroscopic meniscal repair include neurovascular injury, infection, thrombophlebitis, and failure of meniscal healing. Cases of cyst formation and synovitis have also been reported.[56,57]

Neurovascular injuries are among the most common complications of arthroscopic meniscal repair. Saphenous neuropathy has been reported, which patients describe as being only a minor nuisance.[53,58] Peroneal nerve palsy and popliteal artery pseudoaneurysm have also been reported.[59] Detailed knowledge of anatomy, with careful dissection and needle placement, will help in minimizing neurovascular injuries. Surgeon judgment is also of importance, as the use of an all-inside technique for selected posterior horn meniscus tears may be safer than an inside-out repair.

POSTOPERATIVE MANAGEMENT

Immediately after surgery, a compression dressing is applied to the wound, followed by the prescription of ice and elevation of the affected knee to minimize swelling. The knee is immobilized, and crutches are used until quadriceps control is obtained. Patients are seen 1 week postoperatively for a wound assessment and to rule out early complications. Patients are started on an accelerated rehabilitation program and seen at 6 weeks, 3 months, and 6 months postoperatively as needed.

Patients are permitted to weight bear as tolerated, with limited range of motion exercises immediately postoperatively. Knee range of motion is initially restricted from 0° to 90° for the first 6 weeks. During that time, isometric quadriceps exercises are prescribed, and patients are encouraged to use a stationary bike with the seat elevated to avoid deep knee flexion. Time to return to work is variable and dependent on the type of employment. Return to sport typically occurs at 6 months, when the effusion has subsided and knee range of motion is full. Patients who have undergone meniscal repair in conjunction with ACL reconstruction participate in standard rehabilitation for their ACL reconstruction, without weight-bearing squats for 6 weeks.[60,61]

FUTURE CONSIDERATIONS

The use of sutures for meniscal repair have proven to be both efficacious and cost effective, with the vertical mattress repair remaining the gold standard.[62] However, vertical mattress repair does require an accessory incision, is more time consuming, and usually requires an assistant, and there is chance for both needle-stick injuries to the operating team and neurovascular complications.

All-inside techniques have been used with variable success, but comparison of bioabsorbable devices with each other and to inside-out repair have not been conclusive. The most recent data suggest that the biomechanical performance of some fourth-generation all-inside devices is equivalent to that of current suture techniques.[53,63] Of the second- and third-generation devices, the Linvatec Biostinger, Smith & Nephew T-Fix, Bionx Meniscus Arrow, and two Arthrex Darts have been shown to have good initial fixation strength in load to failure that was comparable with that of horizontal mattress suture techniques.[63,64] Only the Bionx Arrow, Linvatec Biostinger, and Clearfix Screw had retained their initial strength through 24 weeks of hydrolysis time.[64] Ultimately, the combination of a simplified surgical technique and high initial clinical healing rates (75%–92%), especially with concomitant ACL reconstruction, and relatively minor complications, made these devices attractive for appropriate meniscal tears.[65] Unfortunately the long-term follow-up showed unacceptably high failure rates, and consequently their use has been largely abandoned.[66]

Future directions for meniscus repair include biologic methods of restoring the meniscus, including the delivery of growth factors or platelet-rich fibrin clot, and transplantation of autogenous fibrochondrocytes into meniscal defects. Other areas of ongoing research include investigation into the use of cytokines to enhance meniscal healing, and the potential to augment meniscal repairs with gene therapy techniques.[67,68]

SUMMARY

The importance of the menisci to knee biomechanics and function have become apparent, and repair of meniscal tears with appropriate characteristics remains the standard. The arthroscopic inside-out suture repair affords a method for stable anatomic reduction and stimulation of circulation, factors that contribute to healing. Repairs by this method have been reported to have a greater than 90% success rate, with a minimum of complications when performed appropriately.

REFERENCES

1. Greis PE, Bardana DD, Holmstrom MC, et al. Meniscal injury: I. Basic science and evaluation. J Am Acad Orthop Surg 2002;10(3):168–76.
2. Petrosini AV, Sherman OH. A historical perspective on meniscal repair. Clin Sports Med 1996;15(3):445–53.
3. Annandale T. An Operation for displaced semilunar cartilage. Br Med J 1885;1(1268): 779.
4. Bland-Sutton J. Ligaments: Their nature and morphology. 2nd edition. London: HK Lewis; 1897.
5. Ikeuchi H. Meniscus surgery using the Watanabe arthroscope. Orthop Clin North Am 1979;10(3):629–42.
6. Newman AP, Daniels AU, Burks RT. Principles and decision making in meniscal surgery. Arthroscopy 1993;9(1):33–51.
7. Fukubayashi TaK, H. The contact area and pressure distribution pattern of the knee. A study of normal and osteoarthrotic knee joints. Acta Orthop Scand 1980;51(6): 871–9.
8. Walker PS, Erkman MJ. The role of the menisci in force transmission across the knee. Clin Orthop Relat Res 1975;(109):184–92.
9. Fairbank TJ. Knee joint changes after meniscectomy. J Bone Joint Surg Br 1948; 30B(4):664–70.
10. Henning CE, Clark JR, Lynch MA, et al. Arthroscopic meniscus repair with a posterior incision. Instr Course Lect 1988;37:209–21.
11. Aglietti P, Zaccherotti G, De Biase P, et al. A comparison between medial meniscus repair, partial meniscectomy, and normal meniscus in anterior cruciate ligament reconstructed knees. Clin Orthop Relat Res 1994;(307):165–73.

12. Johnson RJ, Kettelkamp DB, Clark W, et al. Factors effecting late results after meniscectomy. J Bone Joint Surg Am 1974;56(4):719–29.

13. Ahmed AM, Burke DL. In-vitro measurement of static pressure distribution in synovial joints—Part I: tibial surface of the knee. J Biomech Eng 1983;105(3):216–25.

14. Baratz ME, Fu FH, Mengato R. Meniscal tears: the effect of meniscectomy and of repair on intraarticular contact areas and stress in the human knee. A preliminary report. Am J Sports Med 1986;14(4):270–5.

15. Cox JS, Nye CE, Schaefer WW, et al. The degenerative effects of partial and total resection of the medial meniscus in dogs' knees. Clin Orthop Relat Res 1975;(109): 178–83.

16. Sommerlath K, Gillquist J. The long-term course of various meniscal treatments in anterior cruciate ligament deficient knees. Clin Orthop Relat Res 1992;(283):207–14.

17. Koski JA, Ibarra C, Rodeo SA, et al. Meniscal injury and repair: clinical status. Orthop Clin North Am 2000;31(3):419–36.

18. Rosenberg TD, Scott SM, Coward DB, et al. Arthroscopic meniscal repair evaluated with repeat arthroscopy. Arthroscopy 1986;2(1):14–20.

19. Ahn JH, Wang JH, Oh I. Modified inside-out technique for meniscal repair. Arthroscopy 2004;20 (Suppl 2):178–82.

20. Graf B, Docter T, Clancy W Jr. Arthroscopic meniscal repair. Clin Sports Med 1987;6(3):525–36.

21. Dervin GF, Downing KJ, Keene GC, et al. Failure strengths of suture versus biodegradable arrow for meniscal repair: an in vitro study. Arthroscopy 1997;13(3):296–300.

22. Noyes FR, Barber-Westin SD. Arthroscopic repair of meniscus tears extending into the avascular zone with or without anterior cruciate ligament reconstruction in patients 40 years of age and older. Arthroscopy 2000;16(8):822–9.

23. Cannon WDJ. Arthroscopic meniscal repair. In: McGinty JB, editor. Operative arthroscopy. New York: Raven Press; 1991.

24. DeHaven KE, Lohrer WA, Lovelock JE. Long-term results of open meniscal repair. Am J Sports Med 1995;23(5):524–30.

25. Schmitz MA, Rouse LM Jr, DeHaven KE. The management of meniscal tears in the ACL-deficient knee. Clin Sports Med 1996;15(3):573–93.

26. Orfaly RM, McConkey JP, Regan WD. The fate of meniscal tears after anterior cruciate ligament reconstruction. Clin J Sport Med 1998;8(2):102–5.

27. Fitzgibbons RE, Shelbourne KD. "Aggressive" nontreatment of lateral meniscal tears seen during anterior cruciate ligament reconstruction. Am J Sports Med 1995;23(2): 156–9.

28. Fox JM, Rintz KG, Ferkel RD. Trephination of incomplete meniscal tears. Arthroscopy 1993;9(4):451–55.

29. Shelbourne KD, Rask BP. The sequelae of salvaged nondegenerative peripheral vertical medial meniscus tears with anterior cruciate ligament reconstruction. Arthroscopy 2001;17(3):270–4.

30. Talley MC, Grana WA. Treatment of partial meniscal tears identified during anterior cruciate ligament reconstruction with limited synovial abrasion. Arthroscopy 2000; 16(1):6–10.

31. Mandelbaum BR, Finerman GA, Reicher MA, et al. Magnetic resonance imaging as a tool for evaluation of traumatic knee injuries. Anatomical and pathoanatomical correlations. Am J Sports Med 1986;14(5):361–70.

32. Reicher MA, Hartzman S, Duckwiler GR, et al. Meniscal injuries: detection using MR imaging. Radiology 1986;159(3):753–7.

33. Crues JV III, Ryu R, Morgan FW. Meniscal pathology. The expanding role of magnetic resonance imaging. Clin Orthop Relat Res 1990;(252):80–7.
34. Thompson WO, Thaete FL, Fu FH, et al. Tibial meniscal dynamics using three-dimensional reconstruction of magnetic resonance images. Am J Sports Med 1991;19(3):210–5[discussion: 215–6].
35. Henning CE, Yearout KM, Vequist SW, et al. Use of the fascia sheath coverage and exogenous fibrin clot in the treatment of complex meniscal tears. Am J Sports Med 1991;19(6):626–31.
36. O'Meara PM. Surgical techniques for arthroscopic meniscal repair. Orthop Rev 1993;22(7):781–90.
37. Zhang Z, Arnold JA, Williams T, et al. Repairs by trephination and suturing of longitudinal injuries in the avascular area of the meniscus in goats. Am J Sports Med 1995;23(1):35–41.
38. Zhang Z, Arnold JA. Trephination and suturing of avascular meniscal tears: a clinical study of the trephination procedure. Arthroscopy 1996;12(6):726–31.
39. Perdue PS Jr, Hummer CD III, Colosimo AJ, et al. Meniscal repair: outcomes and clinical follow-up. Arthroscopy 1996;12(6):694–8.
40. Johannsen HV, Fruensgaard S, Holm A, et al. Arthroscopic suture of peripheral meniscal tears. Int Orthop 1988;12(4):287–90.
41. Brown GC, Rosenberg TD, Deffner KT. Inside-out meniscal repair using zone-specific instruments. Am J Knee Surg 1996;9(3):144–50.
42. Cannon WD Jr. Arthroscopic meniscal repair. Inside-out technique and results. Am J Knee Surg 1996;9(3):137–43.
43. Horibe S, Shino K, Nakata K, et al. Second-look arthroscopy after meniscal repair. Review of 132 menisci repaired by an arthroscopic inside-out technique. J Bone Joint Surg Br 1995;77(2):245–9.
44. Horibe S, Shino K, Maeda A, et al. Results of isolated meniscal repair evaluated by second-look arthroscopy. Arthroscopy 1996;12(2):150–5.
45. Rubman MH, Noyes FR, Barber-Westin SD. Arthroscopic repair of meniscal tears that extend into the avascular zone. A review of 198 single and complex tears. Am J Sports Med 1998;26(1):87–95.
46. Spindler KP, McCarty EC, Warren TA, et al. Prospective comparison of arthroscopic medial meniscal repair technique: inside-out suture versus entirely arthroscopic arrows. Am J Sports Med 2003;31(6):929–34.
47. Miller DB Jr. Arthroscopic meniscus repair. Am J Sports Med 1988;16(4):315–20.
48. Cannon WD Jr, Vittori JM. The incidence of healing in arthroscopic meniscal repairs in anterior cruciate ligament-reconstructed knees versus stable knees. Am J Sports Med 1992;20(2):176–81.
49. Ryu RK, Dunbar WH IV. Arthroscopic meniscal repair with two-year follow-up: a clinical review. Arthroscopy 1988;4(3):168–73.
50. Venkatachalam S, Godsiff SP, Harding ML. Review of the clinical results of arthroscopic meniscal repair. Knee 2001;8(2):129–33.
51. Shelbourne KD, Carr DR. Meniscal repair compared with meniscectomy for bucket-handle medial meniscal tears in anterior cruciate ligament-reconstructed knees. Am J Sports Med 2003;31(5):718–23.
52. Hantes ME, Zachos VC, Varitimidis SE, et al. Arthroscopic meniscal repair: a comparative study between three different surgical techniques. Knee Surg Sports Traumatol Arthrosc 2006;14(12):1232–7.
53. Choi NH, Kim TH, Victoroff BN. Comparison of arthroscopic medial meniscal suture repair techniques: inside-out versus all-inside repair. Am J Sports Med 2009;37(11):2144–50.

54. Small NC. Complications in arthroscopic surgery performed by experienced arthroscopists. Arthroscopy 1988;4(3):215–21.
55. Small NC. Complications in arthroscopic meniscal surgery. Clin Sports Med 1990; 9(3):609–17.
56. Choi NH, Kim SJ. Meniscal cyst formation after inside-out meniscal repair. Arthroscopy 2004;20(1):E1–3.
57. Kelly JD IV, Ebrahimpour P. Chondral injury and synovitis after arthroscopic meniscal repair using an outside-in mulberry knot suture technique. Arthroscopy 2004;20(5): e49–52.
58. Austin KS. Complications of arthroscopic meniscal repair. Clin Sports Med 1996; 15(3):613–9.
59. Brasseur P, Sukkarieh F. Iatrogenic pseudo-aneurysm of the popliteal artery. Complication of arthroscopic meniscectomy. Apropos of a case. J Radio. 1990;71(4): 301–4.
60. Buseck MS, Noyes FR. Arthroscopic evaluation of meniscal repairs after anterior cruciate ligament reconstruction and immediate motion. Am J Sports Med 1991; 19(5):489–94.
61. Barber FA, Click SD. Meniscus repair rehabilitation with concurrent anterior cruciate reconstruction. Arthroscopy 1997;13(4):433–7.
62. Rimmer MG, Nawana NS, Keene GC, et al. Failure strengths of different meniscal suturing techniques. Arthroscopy 1995;11(2):146–50.
63. Barber FA, Herbert MA, Richards DP. Load to failure testing of new meniscal repair devices. Arthroscopy 2004;20(1):45–50.
64. Arnoczky SP, Lavagnino M. Tensile fixation strengths of absorbable meniscal repair devices as a function of hydrolysis time. An in vitro experimental study. Am J Sports Med 2001;29(2):118–23.
65. Farng E, Sherman O. Meniscal repair devices: a clinical and biomechanical literature review. Arthroscopy 2004;20(3):273–86.
66. Kurzweil PR, Tifford CD, Ignacio EM. Unsatisfactory clinical results of meniscal repair using the meniscus arrow. Arthroscopy 2005;21(8):905.
67. Ochi M, Uchio Y, Okuda K, et al. Expression of cytokines after meniscal rasping to promote meniscal healing. Arthroscopy 2001;17(7):724–31.
68. Rodeo SA, Warren RF. Meniscal repair using the outside-to-inside technique. Clin Sports Med 1996;15(3):469–81.

Meniscal Repair—Outside-In Repair

Timothy R. Vinyard, MD[a], Brian R. Wolf, MD, MS[a,b,*]

KEYWORDS

- Meniscus • Outside-in • Repair • Arthroscopy
- Knee injury

HISTORICAL PERSPECTIVE

In 1948, Fairbank[1] described the radiographic changes that develop after meniscectomy, suggesting the protective effect of the meniscus. Early biomechanical studies have further defined the importance of the meniscus in normal knee joint function. These studies found a 50% to 70% reduction in femoral condyle contact, a 100% increase in contact stress with removal of the medial meniscus, a 40% to 50% decrease in contact area, and increase in contact stress to 200% to 300% with removal of the lateral meniscus.[2,3] Since then, it has become a well-accepted notion that the menisci play a critical role in load transmission, shock absorption, and secondary stabilization of the knee. Acceptance of the crucial role of the meniscus in knee kinematics coupled with improved understanding of meniscal healing, anatomy, microstructure, and biochemistry has led to the concept that, whenever feasible, the meniscus should be preserved rather than resected.

As the preferred method of treatment of meniscal injuries has swung from resection to preservation over the last several decades, the techniques used to repair meniscal tears has also evolved. Current techniques typically use an arthroscope and favor smaller incisions to decrease the amount of surgical trauma. Techniques are commonly described as outside-in, inside-out, and all-inside, with each technique having it own advantages and disadvantages.

The outside-in technique is named for the direction that the suture is first passed into the knee joint. As described in further detail in the technique section of this report, several subtle technique variations exist when performing an outside-in meniscal repair, but all techniques use a spinal needle to enter the joint under direct visualization, minimizing the risk of injury to both articular cartilage and extracapsular

The authors disclose no conflicts.

[a] Department of Orthopaedic Surgery and Rehabilitation, University of Iowa Hospitals and Clinics, 200 Hawkins Drive, Iowa City, IA 52246, USA
[b] University of Iowa Athletics, 200 Hawkins Drive, Iowa City, IA 52246, USA
* Corresponding author. Department of Orthopaedic Surgery and Rehabilitation, University of Iowa Hospitals and Clinics, 200 Hawkins Drive, Iowa City, IA 52246.
E-mail address: brian-wolf@uiowa.edu

Clin Sports Med 31 (2012) 33–48
doi:10.1016/j.csm.2011.08.011
0278-5919/12/$ – see front matter Published by Elsevier Inc.

neurovascular structures. Unlike the inside-out technique, the outside-in technique does not require the use of a rigid cannula and, therefore, the risk of articular cartilage damage is further reduced. Additionally, the outside-in technique can be accomplished with only a small incision to tie sutures over the capsule, minimizing surgical trauma. In this technique, sutures can be placed in a vertical mattress fashion, which has been shown to have an increased ultimate strength compared with horizontal sutures, arrows, suture anchor devices, and staples.[4–7] This review describes the outside-in technique for meniscal repair in detail, including indications and contraindications, preoperative planning, various techniques, postoperative rehabilitation, complications, and results.

INDICATIONS AND CONTRAINDICATIONS

Before deciding whether to use an outside-in meniscal repair technique, one must first decide whether any meniscal repair is indicated. Several factors must be considered, including location of the tear, the type or pattern of the tear, the quality of the meniscal tissue, chronicity of the tear, patient physiologic age, patient expectations and goals, and stability of the knee when contemplating meniscal repair. Although the decision regarding meniscal repair should be individualized for each patient, one commonly accepted criteria for meniscal repairs includes a complete vertical longitudinal repair greater than 10 mm long, a tear within the peripheral one-third of the meniscus or within 3 to 4 mm of the meniscocapsular junction, an unstable tear that can be displaced by probing, a tear without secondary degeneration or deformity, a tear in an active patient, and a tear associated with concurrent ligamentous instability.[8] Perhaps the most important factor to consider is the location of the tear, because tears closer to the periphery of the meniscus have an increased potential to provide a healing response. Meniscal repair is most likely to be successful for an acute, vertical, longitudinal tear in the vascular periphery of the meniscus in a relatively young patient with a stable knee.

Although both acute and chronic tears may be repaired successfully, it is generally accepted that a higher healing rate exists when meniscal tears are repaired acutely. Henning and colleagues[9] reported higher healing rates in meniscal tears repaired within 8 weeks of injury in knees with concomitant anterior cruciate ligament (ACL) tears.[9] Tenuta and Arciero[10] reported better healing rates of meniscal repairs when they were performed within 19 weeks of injury and also reported improved healing rates when a combined ACL reconstruction was performed.[10]

Several additional studies have also found a higher failure rate of meniscal repairs in ACL-deficient knees and, therefore, concomitant ACL reconstruction is recommended.[11,12] However, Fetzer and colleagues[13] recently reported on the MOON cohort of 1014 ACL reconstructions and found that although 36% of knees had medial meniscal tears and 44% of knees had lateral meniscal tears, only 31% of those medial meniscal tears and 12% of the lateral meniscal tears were deemed repairable at the time of surgery. They did recommend consideration of more aggressive attempts at meniscal preservation, such as implants, advanced repairs to avascular zones, and the use of meniscal scaffold replacements.

Warren[14] first described the arthroscopic outside-in technique primarily as a method to decrease the risk of peroneal nerve injury during lateral meniscal repair as well as other problems encountered at that time with inside-out and open meniscal repair techniques. The outside-in meniscal repair technique has since become an accepted technique for repairing meniscal tears in both the medial and lateral menisci. A key advantage of the outside-in technique is the ability for the surgeon to place needles in an accurate fashion, avoiding injury to surrounding neurovascular structures. Additionally, although repairing anterior horn tears have been nearly impossible, or at the least very difficult, to repair with an inside-out technique, many have found the outside-in technique to be particularly useful for these tears. Successful repair of radial tears of the lateral meniscus in the avascular zone using a fibrin clot and the outside-in technique has been reported.[15] The outside-in technique may also be particularly useful in the small knee joints of young children when attempting to stabilize symptomatic Wrisberg-type discoid menisci, because utilization of the inside-out technique requires cannulas that may place the articular cartilage at undue risk. Delivery of a biologic factor to enhance meniscal healing, such as a fibrin clot, can be performed easily via the outside-in technique. Finally, the surgeon may find the outside-in technique to be valuable for suturing a meniscal replacement, such as an allograft or synthetic scaffold, to the capsule, although a combination of techniques may be necessary. We recommend that the surgeon be comfortable with different techniques.

Although the outside-in technique has many advantages, it is important that the surgeon understands the limitations of the technique as well. Because the suture must be passed through a spinal needle, the initial use of a nonabsorbable braided suture is much more difficult than that of a monofilament suture, such as polydioxanone suture. However, after the preliminary placement of a monofilament suture across the tear, the suture may be easily replaced with a nonabsorbable braided suture as subsequently described in the technique section of this article. We also present a method of solely passing a braided suture across the tear if so desired. Additionally, treating tears of the far posterior horns of the menisci may be suboptimal with the inside-out technique. Van Trommel and coworkers[16] reported a decrease rate of healing on second-look arthroscopy of posterior third meniscal tears treated with the outside-in technique compared with tears in the anterior two-thirds. They reasoned that to avoid the nearby critical neurovascular structures, the sutures must be passed in an oblique fashion across posterior horn meniscal tears, resulting in suboptimal coaptation forces.

PREOPERATIVE PLANNING

When considering surgical treatment for a meniscal tear, the treating surgeon should have an honest and detailed discussion with the patient regarding the risks, benefits, and alternatives inherent to both surgical and nonsurgical treatment. In particular, the patient should be informed that meniscal repair requires significantly more postoperative restrictions than a partial meniscectomy and that often, the decision of whether a tear is repairable cannot be made until the intraoperative evaluation. This may be of particular importance to the athlete that is considering surgical intervention just before or during their season or perhaps to the noncompetitive athlete for assorted employment reasons. A complete and detailed examination of the knee should be performed, paying particular attention to any malalignment or instability. The medial meniscus has been determined to be an important secondary restraint to anterior translation of the tibia with respect to the femur.[17] Therefore, the treating surgeon should evaluate closely for a concomitant ACL tear and discuss reconstruction options with the patient, as failure to reconstruct the ACL may place a meniscal repair at risk and increase the potential for future meniscal tears or other degenerative changes.

TECHNIQUE: OUTSIDE-IN MENISCAL REPAIR

The outside-in technique can be performed with only 18-guage spinal needles, an arthroscopic grasper, and suture material.[6,18,19] Also, meniscal repair kits with

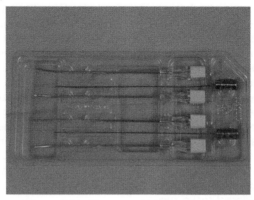

Fig. 1. Several commercially available kits are available, such as the Meniscal Menders (Smith & Nephew, Memphis, TN.)

tailored instruments, such as the Meniscal Mender (Smith and Nephew, Memphis, TN, USA), are commercially available (**Fig. 1**). A nonsterile tourniquet may be placed proximally on the thigh, although it is not typically inflated. The repair may be performed either by dropping the end of the bed and allowing the knee to flex or by keeping the end of the bed straight and allowing the knee to flex by dropping the leg off the side of the operating table. Whichever set up is used, it is important that the leg be positioned so that access is available to the posterior corners both medially and laterally. The joint line may be palpated and marked with a sterile surgical marker to help facilitate accurate needle placement. Other options to enhance accurate needle placement include passing a probe from the contralateral anterior portal over the meniscus at the site of the tear to palpate the tip of the probe from the external skin or to use the arthroscope to transilluminate through the extracapsular tissue as subsequently described in more detail.

As noted previously, the outside-in technique can minimize the risk of damage to neurovascular structures because the entry point of the needle is carefully controlled. When repairing meniscal tears on the lateral side of the knee, needle placement should be anterior to the biceps tendon to avoid injury to the peroneal nerve. The use of curved spinal needles, either commercially available or bent by the surgeon, may be used for far posterior tears to help avoid neurovascular damage. The knee should be maintained at 90° of flexion when repairing lateral meniscal tears to allow the peroneal nerve to fall posteriorly. When the end of the surgical table is kept out straight, the hip may be externally rotated and the knee flexed to place the leg in the "figure of 4" position. This position places the lateral aspect of the knee over the edge of the table, providing access to the posterior aspect of the joint line.

The saphenous nerve and vein are the neurovascular structures on the medial side of the knee that should be avoided when attempting to repair medial meniscal tears. The saphenous nerve becomes subcutaneous approximately 10 cm proximal to the knee joint and branches into its 2 main braches, the infrapatellar and the sartorial branches.[20] The infrapatellar branch of the saphenous nerve is the most commonly injured branch of the saphenous nerve.[20] It crosses over the semitendinosus from its posterior edge and travels anteriorly to provide cutaneous sensation to the antero-lateral aspect of the knee. The semitendinosus can act as an important landmark and can be best palpated with the knee in extension. The infrapatellar branch of the saphenous nerve and vein usually lies anterior to the semitendinosus at the level of the joint line, and keeping the knee in approximately 10° degrees of extension helps to keep the structures anterior to the working area.[18] For tears in the posterior two-thirds of the medial meniscus, the spinal needle should be placed posterior to the semitendinosus tendon to avoid neurovascular damage.[6,18] When repairing an anterior horn tear of the medial meniscus with the outside-in technique, the knee should be positioned in 50° to 60° of flexion, and the spinal needle should enter the joint anterior to the pes anserinus tendons and the saphenous nerve branches.[18] Alternatively, the arthroscope can be placed as far medially as possible within the knee joint and used to produce a wide area of transillumination to clearly demonstrate the saphenous vein.[21] One can then mark the course of the saphenous vein on the skin, recognizing that the saphenous nerve lies just posterior to the vein at this level.[21] Regardless of the location on the knee, we recommend that a small incision and a hemostat or similar device always be utilized to spread down to the joint capsule when tying sutures to avoid entrapment of neurovascular structures.

Standard anteromedial and anterolateral portals are established first. Alternative portals may be established as needed to provide direct access to the tear. It is important to abrade the adjacent surfaces of the tear to remove degenerative tissue that is unlikely to heal and to create a bleeding bed at the site of the tear to help stimulate vascular ingrowth. This may be accomplished with an arthroscopic rasp, a 3.5-mm shaver, or other similar device. Once the synovium and tear have been adequately prepared, the knee is flexed appropriately based on the medial-lateral and anterior-posterior location of the tear. The compartment is further opened by applying a varus or valgus force to the knee when placing the needle. As noted previously, palpation of the joint line and superficial structures aids in placement of the needle. The needle penetrates the meniscus under arthroscopic visualization on either the superior (femoral) or inferior (tibial) surface of the meniscus (**Figs. 2** and **3**). A small probe or small ringed curette may be helpful to provide counter-pressure on the meniscus during needle placement. Additionally, a probe may be helpful to elevate the tip of the needle, especially when placed through the inferior portion of the meniscus to help avoid damage to the articular cartilage surface.

A small incision is made around the first needle puncture and a hemostat is utilized to spread down through the subcutaneous tissues down to the capsule, clearing away small nerves, veins, and tendons from the area at which sutures will be tied (**Fig. 4**). A second spinal needle is introduced through this incision adjacent to the first

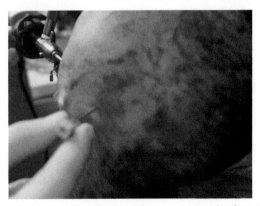

Fig. 2. Percutaneous placement of a spinal needle across a meniscal tear.

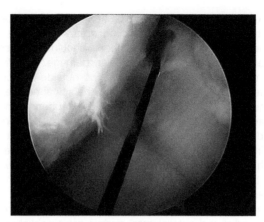

Fig. 3. A monofilament suture is passed into the knee joint.

needle to achieve proper orientation of the sutures depending on tear morphology. We recommend passing both spinal needles across the meniscus before passing suture material to avoid cutting previously placed sutures. A 7-mm cannula may be placed across one of the portals in preparation to pull the sutures out of the knee joint to prevent a soft tissue bridge from becoming caught between the sutures. A rigid, monofilament suture, such as polydioxanone (#0-Polydioxanone, Ethicon; Somerville, NJ, USA) is passed through each spinal needle, grasped within the joint though the previously placed cannula, and generally brought out from the knee anteriorly (**Figs. 5** and **6**) Absorbable sutures are recommended if suture placement requires penetration of the medial collateral ligament, semimembranosus, or popliteal tendon.

The outside-in technique allows for the sutures to be placed in whatever orientation the surgeon deems optimal based on tear morphology. Vertically orientated sutures are likely more effective at grasping the circumferentially oriented collagen fibers of the meniscus, and past studies have found that vertical mattress sutures are more biomechanically sound than horizontal mattress sutures.[5,22–25] Placement of a vertical mattress suture requires that 1 needle be passed across the tear, entering the

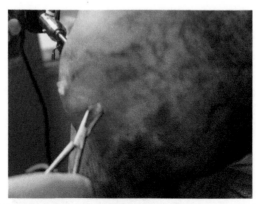

Fig. 4. A small incision is made and a hemostat is used to spread down onto the external capsule.

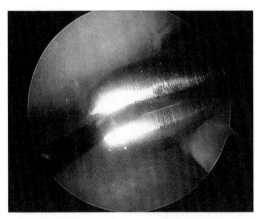

Fig. 5. The suture is grasped within the joint and pulled out through the anterior portal.

superior surface of the meniscus, and the second needle be placed across the synovial junction superior to the meniscus. Placement of horizontal mattress sutures requires that both needles pass through either the superior or inferior side of the meniscus and are tied parallel to the joint line over the capsule. Suture placement may alternate between the superior and inferior meniscal surfaces to evenly approximate the meniscus to the capsule.

Once sutures have been passed across the tear, several technique variations exist for completing the repair. Perhaps the simplest method is to bring the sutures out of the knee joint through a cannula. A knot is then placed at the end of each suture (the so-called "Mulberry knot") with 3 or 4 throws of a standard square-knot fashion, and the ends of each suture are trimmed immediately adjacent to each knot (**Fig. 7**). The sutures are then pulled back flush against the meniscus, bringing the tear into a reduced position (**Fig. 8**). The surgeon can then turn their attention to the external surface of the knee joint and tie the remaining ends of the suture together over the capsule under direct visualization to avoid entrapping neurovascular structures (**Fig. 9**). Each suture placed should be tied individually and inspected before placing additional sutures to avoid suture entanglement.

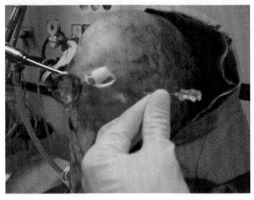

Fig. 6. The ends of the suture sit outside the anterior portal and outside the spinal needle.

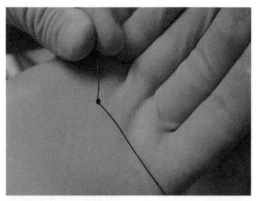

Fig. 7. A Mulberry knot is tied in the suture.

While the above method results in knots on the inside of the knee joint, an alternative method of completing the repair exists in which no knots are left on the inside of the joint. This method entails bringing the 2 ends of the suture that have been passed around the tear outside the knee joint and then tying the 2 ends together. The knot is then pulled through the meniscus to create a single mattress repair across the tear. A small hemostat may be attached to the end of the each suture to prevent inadvertent passage of the end of the suture into the knee joint. The surgeon may find the passage of the knot through the meniscus or capsule somewhat difficult, and the knot can be more easily passed by first tying a "dilator knot" of only 2 throws in front of the larger knot so that the dilator knot first passes through the meniscus. The dilator knot creates a small opening, allowing easier passage of the larger knot. If the sutures are placed in a vertical mattress fashion with 1 suture solely passing through the capsule, then the suture should be shuttled so that the knot passes through the capsule to avoid passing the knot through the meniscus. The surgeon then ties the external ends of the suture onto the capsule under direct visualization.

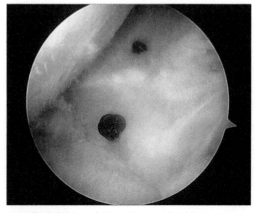

Fig. 8. The sutures are pulled tight, reducing the meniscal tear.

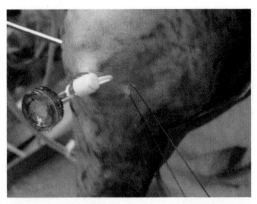

Fig. 9. The monofilament suture strands are ready to be tied onto the capsule under direct visualization.

At least 1 biomechanical study has suggested that, when placed in a vertical mattress fashion, monofilament suture is superior to braided suture.[23] However, if a surgeon desires to replace the monofilament with a braided a suture, a simple additional step is all that is necessary. After placement of the mattress suture across the tear and before tying the free end of the suture on the capsule, a braided suture is tied to the free end of one of the suture strands. Then, by pulling on the opposite end of the monofilament suture, the braided suture replaces the monofilament suture. This can be visualized arthroscopically. The free ends of the braided suture can then be tied over the capsule in the standard fashion.

Finally, a technique exists to completely avoid use of a monofilament suture and is perhaps most easily performed with the use of commercially available products, such as the Meniscal Mender (Smith & Nephew, Memphis, TN, USA). This technique involves passage of a needle near the edge of the meniscal tear and deployment of a wire loop through the needle (**Fig. 10**). A braided suture is then passed into the knee joint through a cannula in an anterior portal using a grasper and then through the open loop (**Fig. 11**). The loop and needle are then withdrawn, pulling one end of the suture

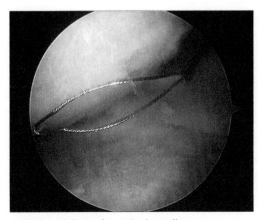

Fig. 10. A wire loop is deployed through a spinal needle.

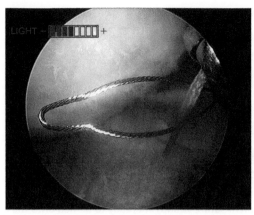

Fig. 11. The braided suture is passed through a cannula and through the open loop.

outside the knee. These basic steps are then essentially repeated, with placement of the needle from outside-in on the opposite side of the meniscal tear. The loop is deployed, and the opposite end of the braided suture is passed into the knee joint, through the cannula and into the loop, which is then pulled out of the knee join to create a knotless suture bridging the meniscal tear (**Fig. 12**). The braided suture is then tied onto the capsule under direct visualization (**Fig. 13**). It is worth noting that the ideal suture material has yet to be definitively determined. As noted, several in vitro biomechanical studies have been performed, and a recent study suggested that suture containing ultra–high-molecular-weight polyethylene may be stronger than braided polyester.[26] However, what, if any, clinical difference exists between various suture materials is unknown.

As noted previously, the outside-in technique is particularly useful for repair of anterior and middle third meniscal tears.[18] To avoid damage to posterior neurovascular structures when attempting to repair posterior horn meniscal tears, curved spinal needles may be utilized. Additionally, the knee may be placed in extension before tying the sutures to help reduce the meniscus to the capsule and prevent

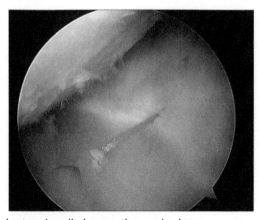

Fig. 12. The braided suture is pulled across the meniscal tear.

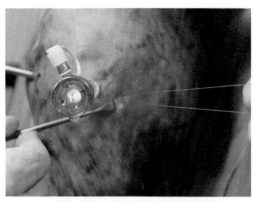

Fig. 13. The braided suture ends are tied down onto the capsule under direct visualization.

entrapment of the posterior capsule that might result in a flexion contracture. If the surgeon finds that using the outside-in technique for posterior horn tears results in suboptimal orientation of the of the sutures across the repair, we recommend considering the outside-in or all-inside techniques for these repairs.

Special technical considerations should be used for particular tear types. For tears associated with ACL reconstruction, we recommend placing the meniscal repair sutures before proceeding with the reconstruction but not tying the sutures until the ACL graft has been secured. Others may prefer to fully complete the repair before constructing the ACL. For large, bucket-handle tears, the displaced fragment should be reduced using a probe or skewering the meniscus with a single needle. The initial suture should be placed at the midpoint of the bucket handle fragment, essentially creating two separate tears. Additional sutures are then placed in an alternating fashion on either side of the original suture until the fragment is evenly opposed to the peripheral portion of the tear. A probe may be particularly useful in holding the bucket-handle fragment in a reduced position while passing needles in an outside-in technique.

POSTOPERATIVE MANAGEMENT

The ideal postoperative rehabilitation protocol after meniscal repair continues to be an area of debate. The tear pattern, any concomitant knee injuries, and the individual patient must be considered when evaluating factors such as weight bearing, range of motion, and return to sport. Although initial meniscal repairs were rehabilitated in a conservative manner, improved understanding of meniscal healing has led many to advocate more accelerated protocols.[27–29] In a dog model, Klein and colleagues[30,31] demonstrated the atrophy of meniscus, ligaments, and bone resulting from immobilizations and non–weight bearing that was prevented when active range of motion was added to the non–weight bearing protocol. Dowdy and coworkers[32] reported diminished collagen content within the healing meniscus after prolonged immobilization after meniscal repair in a dog model. However, Anderson and colleagues[33] used a sheep model to show that the tensile properties of the meniscus were not significantly affected if only limited motion was permitted. The results of these studies suggest that it is beneficial to include range of motion of the knee after isolated meniscal repair. Alternatively, Guisasola and colleagues[34] found no significant difference between immobilization and early motion 6 weeks after surgery in a sheep model.

Although clinical studies have shown good rates of meniscal healing using accelerated rehabilitation protocols, an important limitation of these studies is that meniscal healing was evaluated only on the basis of patient-reported symptoms.[27–29] Furthermore, it has been reported that tears may be asymptomatic despite having only partial healing.[16] The importance of complete healing was suggested in a study by Asahina and coworkers[35] in which patients with incompletely healed meniscal tears with second-look arthroscopy required additional meniscal surgery at a rate almost 5 times higher than those that with completely healed meniscal tears.

Meniscal tear pattern may help to guide decisions regarding rehabilitation after meniscal repair. For vertical, longitudinal tears, weight bearing in extension appears to be safe, because, based on multiple studies, it is generally accepted that compressive loads applied with the knee in extension reduce the torn fragment to the periphery of the knee. Conversely, others have reported that weight bearing with the knee in flexion causes the posterior horn to displace from the capsule.[36,37] Compressive loads in extension placed across radial tears may be expected to increase hoop stresses and the stress across the repair.[18] Therefore, it may be advisable to limit early weight bearing after repair of a radial tear. Additionally, Thompson and coworkers[38] found that the meniscus translates posteriorly with knee flexion, but only minimal translation occurred at flexion angles less than 60°. Thus, limitation of extreme flexion during the early phases of meniscal healing should be considered.

Our preferred rehabilitation protocol includes placing the patient in a hinged brace for 6 weeks postoperatively. For the first 4 weeks, the patient is allowed to bear weight as tolerated with crutches with the expectation that they will slowly wean themselves off of the crutches after 7 to 14 days. The brace is to be locked in extension when they are ambulating, but they are able to range their knee from 0° to 90°. Therapeutic exercises include passive range of motion to tolerance; patella mobilization; quadriceps, hamstring, and gluteal sets; hamstring stretches; hip strengthening; and straight leg raises. For weeks 4 to 6, we allow the patient to increase their range of motion when ambulating to 0° to 90°. When not ambulating, they may range their knee from 0° to 120°. Therapeutic exercises are advanced to include stationary biking when flexion reaches 110°. We ask that the patient avoid twisting while weight bearing and avoid squatting beyond 90°. Weeks 6 through 12 include weaning the patient completely from the brace and progression to full, pain-free range of motion. Additional therapeutic exercises include proprioception training, foot work, and closed kinetic chain exercises. Weeks 12 through 16 include the addition of light jogging and the gradual progression to sport-specific training if all symptoms have resolved and full range of motion has been obtained. After repair of isolated radial split tears of the lateral meniscus or more complex tears, toe-touch weight bearing is recommended for 2 to 4 weeks with the knee locked in extension. The rehabilitation protocol is modified because of the increased lateral meniscal excursion observed with flexion. Weight bearing, range of motion, and strengthening are progressively advanced after the first 4 weeks.

COMPLICATIONS

Fortunately, complications specific to meniscal repair are rare and can be minimized when careful attention is paid to technique and local anatomy. When complications do occur, they tend involve damage to nerve or vascular structures, stiffness, or failure of the meniscus to heal. As noted previously, the saphenous nerve is at risk with medial meniscal repairs, either when placing needles into the joint or when tying sutures down onto the capsule. Injury to the saphenous nerve can be minimized by paying careful attention to anatomic landmarks, transillumination of the saphenous vein, and by dissecting down onto the capsule before tying sutures. The peroneal nerve is at risk when repairing lateral meniscal tears. Placing the knee at 90° of flexion and keeping the needle entry points anterior to the biceps femoris tendon minimize this risk. The posterior neurovascular structures are at risk when attempting to repair posterior horn meniscal tears. Curved needles may help minimize this risk but may also lead to the placement of sutures in an oblique orientation across the tear, which is suboptimal from a biomechanical standpoint. The inside-out technique or all-inside technique may be more appropriate for these posterior tears. In theory, entrapment of the posterior capsule leading to loss of full extension can occur if the knee is held in too much flexion when the sutures are passing through the posterior capsule are tied, especially on the medial side. However, if the knee is held near full extension with a valgus force applied to the knee, which reduces the capsule to the meniscus, this risk is minimized. Meniscal repairs can fail for many reasons, but the most common causes include poor indications for repair, such as inadequate vascular supply or degenerative tissue; poor surgical technique, such as oblique orientation of suture across a tear; inadequate protection of the repair; unrecognized or untreated instability of the knee; or re-injury. Careful attention to proper patient selection, repair technique, and rehabilitation protocol can minimize failures.

RESULTS

Although there are relatively few studies evaluating the results of the outside-in meniscal repair technique, most show a high rate of healing with excellent clinical results. Morgan and Casscells[39] have been credited with the first report of the outside-in technique and found excellent clinical results in 98.6% of 70 patients with posterior horn tears. Their results were based solely on clinical evaluation, and their only reported complications were a transient saphenous nerve irritation and 1 case of deep infection. Morgan and coworkers[36] would later report on 353 meniscal tears repaired through the outside-in approach. Second-look arthroscopy was performed on 74 repairs with an overall asymptomatic healing rate of 84%. Sixty-five percent were completely healed, and 19% were incompletely healed. Interestingly, all of the failures were in knees that were ACL deficient, and all tears were located in the posterior horns. No failures occurred in the ACL uninjured knees or in the ACL reconstructed group, and visual evidence of healing requires a 4-month time interval.

Mariani and colleagues[29] reported the results of meniscal tears treated with the outside-in technique with concomitant ACL reconstruction in 22 patients. These patients also underwent what was considered an accelerated rehabilitation program at that time, including immediate range of motion and weight-bearing. Outcome measures included clinical evaluations and magnetic resonance imaging which found 77.3% good clinical results with only 3 patients having clinical signs of meniscal retear.

Van Trommel and colleagues[16] showed healing rates that varied according to the region of the repair when using the outside-in technique. Patients were evaluated at an average of 15 months after surgery with second-look arthroscopy, arthrography, or magnetic resonance imaging. Seventy-six percent showed complete or partial healing with 24% having no healing. Significantly lower healing rates were noted in tears of the posterior horn of the medial meniscus, and in all 15 patients who had tears extending from the posterior third to the middle third of the medial meniscus that were partially healed, it was always the posterior third that did not heal. As noted previously, the authors reasoned that oblique placement of suture through the meniscus leads to suboptimal coaptation forces resulting in decreased healing rates. In a more recent study, Yiannakopoulos and coworkers[40] described their modification of the outside-in technique and reported their results in 8 patients. The meniscus repair took an average of 11 minutes and at a follow-up between 6 to 14 months, no patients reported symptoms consistent with meniscal tear. Second-look arthroscopy was performed in 1 patient with complete healing noted.

In perhaps the only study comparing the outside-in technique, the inside-out technique, and the all-inside technique, Hantes and colleagues[41] evaluated 57 patients undergoing meniscal repair at a mean of 22 months' follow-up. The criteria for clinical success included absence of joint line tenderness, locking, swelling, and a negative McMurray test. Seventeen of the 57 patients were treated with the outside-in technique and a 100% healing rate was reported in this group, compared with a 95% healing rate for the inside-out technique and a 65% healing rate for the all-inside cohort. However, the time required for the repair averaged 38.5 minutes in the outside-in group, 18.1 minutes for the inside-out group, and 13.6 minutes for the all-inside group. Only 1 patient from the outside-in repair group had a transient saphenous nerve palsy, compared with 3 patients in the inside-out group. All patients had complete resolution of their symptoms by 4 months after surgery.

SUMMARY

When treating meniscal tears that have been deemed repairable, the outside-in technique is an effective and safe method of repair. Damage to neurovascular structures and articular cartilage, which may be seen with other techniques, is theoretically minimized by thorough knowledge of pertinent anatomy and accurate placement of needles. Repair can be achieved with minimal instruments and is particularly well suited for tears of the anterior horn and midbody. The technique may also be well suited for radial split tears, meniscal allografts, and synthetic meniscal replacements but may be limited in its use for posterior horn tears. A comprehensive rehabilitation should be individualized based on the tear morphology and location as well as any concomitant procedures. Excellent results have been reported that meet or exceed the results of the outside-in and all-inside techniques with minimal complications.

REFERENCES

1. Fairbank TJ. Knee joint changes after meniscectomy. J Bone Joint Surg 1948;30B(4): 664–70.
2. Fukubayashi T, Kurosawa H. The contact area and pressure distribution pattern of the knee. A study of normal and osteoarthrotic knee joints. Acta Orthop 1980;51(6): 871–9.
3. Kettelkamp DB, Jacobs AW. Tibiofemoral contact area—determination and implications. J Bone Joint Surg Am 1972;54(2):349–56.
4. Barber FA, Herbert MA, Richards DP. Load to failure testing of new meniscal repair devices. Arthroscopy 2004;20(1):45–50.
5. Rankin CC, Lintner DM, Noble PC, et al. A biomechanical analysis of meniscal repair techniques. Am J Sports Med 2002;30(4):492–7.
6. Rodeo SA. Arthroscopic meniscal repair with use of the outside-in technique. Instructional Course Lectures 2000;49:195–206.
7. Walsh SP, Evans SL, O'Doherty DM, et al. Failure strengths of suture vs. biodegradable arrow and staple for meniscal repair: an in vitro study. Knee 2001;8(2):151–6.
8. Greis PE, Bardana DD, Holmstrom MC, et al. Meniscal injury: I. Basic science and evaluation. J Am Acad Orthop Surg 2002;10(3):168–76.
9. Henning CE, Lynch MA, Yearout KM, et al. Arthroscopic meniscal repair using an exogenous fibrin clot. Clin Orthop Relat Res 1990;(252):64–72.

10. Tenuta JJ, Arciero RA. Arthroscopic evaluation of meniscal repairs. Factors that effect healing. Am J Sports Med 1994;22(6):797–802.
11. Cooper DE, Arnoczky SP, Warren RF. Arthroscopic meniscal repair. Clin Sports Med 1990;9(3):589–607.
12. Warren RF. Meniscectomy and repair in the anterior cruciate ligament-deficient patient. Clin Orthop Relat Res 1990;(252):55–63.
13. Fetzer GB, Spindler KP, Amendola A, et al. Potential market for new meniscus repair strategies: evaluation of the MOON cohort. J Knee Surg 2009;22(3):180–6.
14. Warren RF. Arthroscopic meniscus repair. Arthroscopy 1985;1(3):170–2.
15. van Trommel MF, Simonian PT, Potter HG, et al. Arthroscopic meniscal repair with fibrin clot of complete radial tears of the lateral meniscus in the avascular zone. Arthroscopy 1998;14(4):360–5.
16. van Trommel MF, Simonian PT, Potter HG, et al. Different regional healing rates with the outside-in technique for meniscal repair. Am J Sports Med 1998;26(3):446–52.
17. Levy IM, Torzilli PA, Warren RF. The effect of medial meniscectomy on anterior-posterior motion of the knee. J Bone Joint Surg Am 1982;64(6):883–8.
18. Wolf BR, Cohen DB, Rodeo SA. Outside-in meniscal repair. Techniques in knee surgery. 2004;3(1):19–28.
19. Rodeo SA, Warren RF. Meniscal repair using the outside-to-inside technique. Clin Sports Med 1996;15(3):469–81.
20. Kim TK, Savino RM, McFarland EG, et al. Neurovascular complications of knee arthroscopy. Am J Sports Med 2002;30(4):619–29.
21. Kelly M, Macnicol MF. Identification of the saphenous nerve at arthroscopy. Arthroscopy 2003;19(5):E46.
22. Kohn D, Siebert W. Meniscus suture techniques: a comparative biomechanical cadaver study. Arthroscopy 1989;5(4):324–7.
23. Post WR, Akers SR, Kish V. Load to failure of common meniscal repair techniques: effects of suture technique and suture material. Arthroscopy 1997;13(6):731–6.
24. Rimmer MG, Nawana NS, Keene GC, et al. Failure strengths of different meniscal suturing techniques. Arthroscopy 1995;11(2):146–50.
25. Asik M, Sener N. Failure strength of repair devices versus meniscus suturing techniques. Knee Surg Sports Traumatol Arthrosc 2002;10(1):25–9.
26. Barber FA, Herbert MA, Schroeder FA, et al. Biomechanical testing of new meniscal repair techniques containing ultra high-molecular weight polyethylene suture. Arthroscopy 2009;25(9):959–67.
27. Barber FA. Accelerated rehabilitation for meniscus repairs. Arthroscopy 1994;10(2):206–10.
28. Barber FA, Click SD. Meniscus repair rehabilitation with concurrent anterior cruciate reconstruction. Arthroscopy 1997;13(4):433–7.
29. Mariani PP, Santori N, Adriani E, et al. Accelerated rehabilitation after arthroscopic meniscal repair: a clinical and magnetic resonance imaging evaluation. Arthroscopy 1996;12(6):680–6.
30. Klein L, Heiple KG, Torzilli PA, et al. Prevention of ligament and meniscus atrophy by active joint motion in a non-weight-bearing model. J Orthop Res 1989;7(1):80–5.
31. Klein L, Player JS, Heiple KG, et al. Isotopic evidence for resorption of soft tissues and bone in immobilized dogs. J Bone Joint Surg Am 1982;64(2):225–30.
32. Dowdy PA, Miniaci A, Arnoczky SP, et al. The effect of cast immobilization on meniscal healing. An experimental study in the dog. Am J Sports Med 1995;23(6):721–8.
33. Anderson DR, Gershuni DH, Nakhostine M, et al. The effects of non-weight-bearing and limited motion on the tensile properties of the meniscus. Arthroscopy 1993;9(4):440–5.

34. Guisasola I, Vaquero J, Forriol F. Knee immobilization on meniscal healing after suture: an experimental study in sheep. Clin Orthop Relat Res 2002;(395):227–33.
35. Asahina S, Muneta T, Hoshino A, et al. Intermediate-term results of meniscal repair in anterior cruciate ligament-reconstructed knees. Am J Sports Med 1998;26(5):688–91.
36. Morgan CD, Wojtys EM, Casscells CD, et al. Arthroscopic meniscal repair evaluated by second-look arthroscopy. Am J Sports Med 1991;19(6):632–7 [discussion: 637–8].
37. Walker PS, Erkman MJ. The role of the menisci in force transmission across the knee. Clin Orthop Relat Res 1975;(109):184–92.
38. Thompson WO, Thaete FL, Fu FH, et al. Tibial meniscal dynamics using three-dimensional reconstruction of magnetic resonance images. Am J Sports Med 1991; 19(3):210–15 [discussion: 215–6].
39. Morgan CD, Casscells SW. Arthroscopic meniscus repair: a safe approach to the posterior horns. Arthroscopy 1986;2(1):3–12.
40. Yiannakopoulos CK, Chiotis I, Karabalis C, et al. A simplified arthroscopic outside-in meniscus repair technique. Arthroscopy 2004;20(Suppl 2):183–6.
41. Hantes ME, Zachos VC, Varitimidis SE, et al. Arthroscopic meniscal repair: a comparative study between three different surgical techniques. Knee Surg Sports Traumatol Arthrosc 2006;14(12):1232–7.

Meniscal Repair with the Newest Fixators—Which are Best?

Eric D. Bava, MD*, F. Alan Barber, MD

KEYWORDS
- Meniscus repair • Suture • Fast-fix • Rapidloc
- OmniSpan • Sequent • Cinch

The meniscus serves several key functions in the human knee. These include contributing to the mechanics of joint lubrication, stability, congruence, and proprioception as well as dispersing the loads across the articular cartilage surfaces.[1–3] The meniscus is especially important for an anterior cruciate ligament (ACL)-deficient knee because it serves as a secondary restraint to anterior tibial translation and protects the knee from arthritic change.[4] The knee undergoes a natural progression of degenerative changes following meniscectomy, as classically described by Fairbank.[5] It is for these reasons that surgical repair of meniscus tears is so important. Unfortunately, most meniscus tears are not amenable to repair and instead result in a partial meniscectomy, making it one of the most commonly performed orthopedic procedures.

Meniscus repair is performed using various techniques and devices. These include outside-in, inside-out, and all-inside repairs as well as "hybrid repairs" that incorporate a combination of both suture and meniscal device repair techniques. Meniscal repair has evolved over time. Initially, a torn meniscus was repaired using an open technique as first reported by Annandale in 1885.[6] It was not until the early 1980s that open meniscal repair techniques were replaced by arthroscopic approaches that provided access to the difficult-to-reach areas of the meniscus and also minimized the risks associated with open surgery, including neurovascular injury. Henning and others pioneered arthroscopic meniscal repair using an inside-out suture repair technique.[7–9] Later, an outside-in meniscus repair technique was developed in order to decrease the risk of injury to the posterior neurovascular structures.[10,11] Recent technological advances have allowed for the development of all-inside meniscus

No funding was received related to the material presented here. Financial disclosure: The authors have received meniscal repair devices for testing and/or research support from the following companies: Arthrex, ConMed Linvatec, DePuy-Mitek, Cayenne Medical, Smith & Nephew Endoscopy, and Biomet Sports Medicine.
Plano Orthopedic Sports Medicine and Spine Center, 5228 West Plano Parkway, Plano, TX 75093, USA
* Corresponding author.

repair techniques[12] that avoid additional incisions, protect the posterior neurovascular elements, and reduce surgical time.

THE MENISCUS AND CONSIDERATIONS FOR REPAIR

Human menisci are crescent-shaped fibrocartilaginous structures with triangular cross sections that are located within both the medial and lateral compartments of the knee. Each meniscus has an anterior and posterior horn and is attached at its periphery to the joint capsule by the coronary ligaments. The blood supply to the meniscus comes from the periphery,[13] and therefore the meniscus periphery is more vascularized and the central portion of the meniscus is avascular. This is important in considering repair of a torn meniscus because in order for a meniscus repair to successfully heal it must have a good vascular supply. The meniscus is divided into 3 zones based on vascularity. The peripheral third of the meniscus is the most vascular and is called the "red/red zone." Blood vessels are found throughout this region. The less vascular middle third is called the "red/white zone." This is the transition area between the well-vascularized "red/red zone" and the avascular inner third of the meniscus, which is called the "white/white zone."[13,14]

The meniscus acts as a shock absorber by deepening the articular surfaces of the tibial plateau, better conforming to the shape of the femoral condyles, and thus increasing the surface area of load distribution.[1–3] This increased surface area allows for lower overall contact stresses. The meniscus converts vertically oriented compression stresses into radially oriented hoop stresses. The meniscus also functions as a secondary stabilizer to the knee joint because it increases the conformity of the distal femur and proximal tibia, which can be important in a knee with ligamentous deficiency. Furthermore, by maintaining space between the femur and tibia, the meniscus allows for better diffusion of synovial fluid within the joint space, and thus provides nutrition and lubrication to the articular cartilage.

Because of the relative avascularity of the meniscus, a torn meniscus rarely has the ability to heal spontaneously and may lack the ability to heal altogether. Two factors that play a key role in healing potential are tear pattern and location. Meniscus tears can be classified as radial, horizontal, and longitudinal (bucket-handle). Complex tears occur when a combination of these patterns exist. Careful evaluation of the meniscus tear is necessary in order to correctly recognize the tear pattern and determine its ability for repair. Tear location is important because this determines the healing capacity of a meniscus repair. Meniscus tears that are within 3 mm from the meniscosynovial junction (within the "red/red zone") are considered vascular and are more likely to heal. Tears that are located 3 to 5 mm from the meniscosynovial junction (within the "red/white zone") can have variable vascularity,[13,14] and those tears that occur over 5 mm from the meniscosynovial junction (within the "white/white zone") are usually considered avascular.

The poor vascularity of the meniscus may lead to a decreased likelihood of healing in a meniscal repair. Therefore, it is important to use techniques that optimize the healing environment. This can be done with good tissue preparation along with appropriate meniscus fixation. Rasping of both torn edges of the meniscus and the perimeniscal synovium above and below the meniscus helps stimulate a healing response.[15,16] Also, vascular access channels may be created through trephination of the meniscus with an 18-gauge (or larger) spinal needle. This can result in fibrovascular healing in avascular areas of the meniscus.[17] The addition of a fibrin clot[8,18] or platelet-rich fibrin matrix[19] to the tear site has also been suggested to aid healing of a torn meniscus.

Fixation strength and time are 2 final important factors to consider for successful repair of a torn meniscus. Although the forces within the knee can be as high as 4 times body weight with normal gait,[20] it appears that the meniscus experiences only compressive, not distractive, forces during normal unloaded knee motion.[21–23] This suggests that the fixation used for meniscal repair functions by maintaining the alignment of the meniscus tissue while healing occurs and avoiding sheer stresses, rather than resisting distractive forces. Meniscal healing occurs with time and studies have indicated that meniscus repairs can be considerably weaker at the meniscal repair scar even after 12 weeks.[24] Morgan and colleagues noted that about 4 months was required in order for meniscal repairs to demonstrate visual evidence of meniscus healing on second-look arthroscopy.[25]

SURGICAL TECHNIQUES OF MENISCUS FIXATION

Arthroscopic techniques have almost completely replaced open meniscal repair techniques. These arthroscopic techniques include arthroscopically assisted inside-out and outside-in repairs that require accessory incisions to be made. Alternatively, completely arthroscopic "all-inside" meniscus repairs using recently developed meniscal repair devices do not require an accessory incision. Several generations of "all-inside" meniscal repair device designs have been developed. These include both rigid implants and suture-based fixators. For all suture-based repairs, vertically oriented nonabsorbable sutures are considered to be the gold standard because of the high failure loads[26] they provide. This is because with vertically oriented sutures, the suture loop captures the strong circumferential fibers of the meniscus.

Inside-Out Repair

In order to perform an inside-out meniscal suture repair, nonabsorbable sutures attached at each end of 2 long flexible needles are placed through the meniscus tissue with the use of curved cannulas. Using arthroscopic visualization, curved cannulas of varying angles are placed through an arthroscopic portal. The cannula is used to direct the flexible needles into the torn portion of the meniscus, allowing for either a horizontal or vertical suture pattern. Once each needle is passed through the meniscus periphery, it is identified outside of the joint capsule through a small incision. The needles are retrieved through the incision and the attached corresponding sutures are tied over the joint capsule. Through the incision, the neurovascular structures at risk can be retracted out of the field and thus injury can be avoided. The varying angles of the cannulas allow for access to the anterior, middle, and posterior regions of the meniscus[27,28] and therefore the inside-out repair is appropriate for all meniscal tears.

Outside-In Repair

An outside-in suture repair can be useful for tears in the anterior and middle thirds of the meniscus,[29] and several variations of the technique exist. To perform this repair technique, a large gauge needle is placed percutaneously under arthroscopic guidance, through the peripheral meniscus rim and inner torn portion of the meniscus. Through the lumen of the needle a monofilament suture can be passed and retrieved from within the joint space. With one variation, the suture is retrieved by a small metal snare that is passed through a second percutaneously placed needle. The corresponding suture ends are tied over the joint capsule through a small accessory incision. With another variation of this technique the suture is retrieved through an anterior arthroscopy portal and multiple knots ("mulberry knot") are tied on the end of the suture.[10,11] When the suture end is tensioned, the knot is drawn against the meniscus within the joint and acts as an anchor that draws the meniscus fragment against the meniscal rim. One advantage of the outside-in technique is that the accessory incision can be smaller than what is usually necessary for an inside-out repair. However, outside-in repair techniques are not appropriate for tears of the posterior horn because of the risk to neurovascular structures.[30]

All-Inside Repair

All-inside meniscus repairs are performed solely through arthroscopic portals, avoid the need for accessory incisions, and decrease the risk of neurovascular injury. This technique uses various meniscal repair devices and is best suited for tears within the posterior horn of the meniscus. The meniscal repair devices can be either rigid implants or self-adjusting suture-based implants. The first generation designs for all-inside meniscus repair systems consisted of small rigid, mostly absorbable implants that secured the torn portion of the meniscus to the peripheral rim. The newest generation of all-inside meniscal repair devices use suture to secure the torn inner portion of the meniscus to the outer meniscus rim. These self-adjusting suture-based designs have incorporated advances in suture materials (ultra high molecular weight polyethylene [UHMWPE]-containing suture) and newer polymers used in suture anchors.

FIRST-GENERATION DEVICES (RIGID IMPLANTS)

The first generation of all-inside meniscal repair devices were usually rigid or semirigid devices contained barbs or screw threads and provided meniscal fixation by piercing the meniscal fragment and meniscus rim and thus spanning the tear site. These devices were inserted perpendicular to the tear and required adequate meniscus tissue on both sides of the tear for good purchase. These devices were usually made of bioabsorbable polymers such as poly-L-lactic acid (PLLA) and were intended to have a low profile on the meniscus surface in order to minimize the risk of articular cartilage abrasion.[31]

A number of different designs have been developed including tacks, staples, and screws. Tack devices gained wide use initially and the first tack was the Meniscus Arrow (ConMed Linvatec, Largo, FL, USA). Later modifications of this device led to a reduced profile and more rapid rate of degradation in the Contour Arrow. Other designs include the Meniscal Dart (Arthrex, Naples, FL, USA) with a double reverse barb pattern and the BioStinger (ConMed Linvatec, Largo, FL, USA), which has 4 rows of barbs for tissue fixation and a low-profile head that can be countersunk to sit just below the meniscal surface. The meniscus staple works similar to tacks, although it has 2 tacks spanned by a suture to repair the meniscal tear. This device has been called the PolySorb meniscal staple (United States Surgical, North Haven, CT, USA), and the SDsorb staple (Surgical Dynamics, Norwalk, CT, USA). The Biomet meniscal staple (Biomet, Warsaw, IN, USA) was a rigid device without a spanning suture and is no longer available. Meniscal screw designs seek to gain purchase in both segments of the meniscus and span the tear site with compressive screw threads. These include the Meniscal Screw (Biomet, Warsaw, IN, USA), the Clearfix Meniscal Screw (Mitek, Raynham, MA, USA), and the Trinion Screw (Inion Ltd, Tampere, Finland). In addition, the Mitek Meniscal Repair System (Mitek, Raynham, MA, USA) is an "H-shaped" molded polymer device that uses a single curved shaft connecting 2 perpendicular cross bars for meniscus fixation.

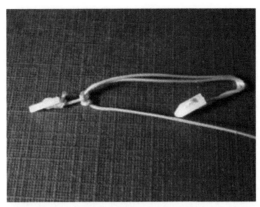

Fig. 1. The FasT-Fix consisted of two 5-mm PLLA or polyacetal anchors connected with a preloaded, pre-tied, self-sliding, and self-locking knot of No. 0 nonabsorbable braided polyester suture. (*Courtesy of* F. A. Barber MD, Plano, TX.)

SELF-ADJUSTING SUTURE CONTAINING IMPLANTS

The newest generation is all-inside self-adjusting meniscal repair devices that deliver a nonabsorbable UHMWPE-containing suture across the meniscus repair site in a completely arthroscopic manner. These devices generally consist of nonabsorbable anchors that are connected by suture with pre-tied, sliding, and self-locking knot. The insertion devices are placed through an anterior arthroscopic portal and the anchors are then passed through the meniscal fragment and peripheral rim. Once the anchor is deployed it is located extra-articularly on the capsular surface. Once deployed, the sliding-locking knot in the suture can be cinched in order to compress the meniscal repair site. These devices allow for flexible fixation of meniscal fragments and may potentially allow for either horizontal or vertical suture configurations.

The FasT-Fix (Smith & Nephew, Andover, MA, USA) was the first of the all-inside self-adjusting suture devices (**Fig. 1**). It consisted of two 5-mm anchors, made of either PLLA (absorbable) or polyacetal (nonabsorbable) material, which were connected by a No. 0, nonabsorbable braided polyester suture. The anchors were delivered via a 16.5-gauge arthroscopic insertion needle that was either straight or angled 22°. Once both anchors were securely placed, the pre-tied sliding-locking knot was tensioned by pulling the free suture end taut while a knot pusher/suture cutter slid down the suture tail. Once tensioned, the free suture end was then cut. The original Fast-Fix was subsequently modified in several ways. The insertion needle was reconfigured to facilitate insertion and later the braided polyester suture was replaced with No. 0 UHMWPE suture (UltraBraid), making the repair stronger and the suture less likely to break. The device was renamed the Ultra Fast-Fix and represented a significant advance over the earlier version. The latest iteration of the FasT-Fix is called the FasT-Fix 360. It has 2 poly ether ether ketone (PEEK) anchors connected with No. 0 UltraBraid suture, which has a sliding locking knot. The single round handle has a curved needle (**Fig. 2**). As of the time of this writing, this device is in the process of being released. Preliminary testing and an examination of the prototype suggest it will represent another substantial upgrade of this meniscal repair device system.

Following release of the FasT-Fix, the RapidLoc (Mitek, Raynham, MA, USA) became commercially available (**Fig. 3**). This device consists of a PLLA "backstop" soft-tissue anchor, which is attached by either a No. 2-0 absorbable Panacryl suture

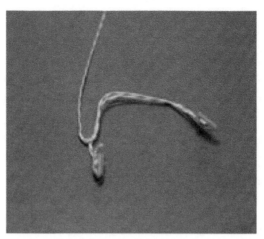

Fig. 2. The FasT-Fix 360 has 2 PEEK anchors connected with No. 0 UltraBraid suture, which has a sliding locking knot inserted using a round-handled device with a curved needle. (*Courtesy of* F. A. Barber MD, Plano, TX.)

or nonabsorbable braided polyester suture to a PLLA or PDS (polydioxanone) "top hat." The absorbable Panacryl suture was associated with the PDS "top hat" in the device. The "backstop" anchor is inserted across the meniscus tear into an extracapsular position using a gun that has a needle "barrel." This needle is provided in straight, angled 12°, or angled 27° versions. As the suture is tensioned, the pre-tied sliding knot and "top hat" are advanced securely against the superior surface of the meniscus, compressing the meniscus repair site and causing the "top hat" to dimple the meniscus surface.

The RapidLoc device has been recently replaced by a newer version called the OmniSpan (**Fig. 4**). This revision is a significant change from the original form. Instead of using a single suture, a loop of No. 0 OrthoCord (a combination of 55% PDS and 45% UHMWPE) is woven between 2 PEEK anchors in a loop. A sliding locking knot

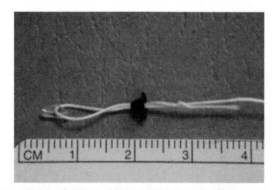

Fig. 3. The RapidLoc consists of a 5 mm × 1.5 mm "backstop" soft-tissue anchor, a connecting suture of either No. 2-0 absorbable Panacryl or No. 2-0 nonabsorbable braided polyester suture, and a PLLA or PDS (polydioxanone) "top hat." (*Courtesy of* F. A. Barber MD, Plano, TX.)

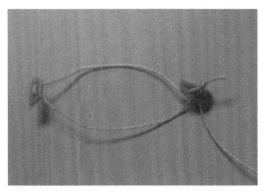

Fig. 4. OmniSpan is the current revision of the previous RapidLoc. It has a loop of No. 0 OrthoCord woven between 2 PEEK anchors with a sliding locking knot located outside the first deployed anchor. (*Courtesy of* F. A. Barber MD, Plano, TX.)

is located on the outside of the loop reinforcing the first anchor to be deployed. Consequently when deployed, a double suture repair spans the repair site in either a vertical or horizontal mattress configuration. As the single suture extending out the arthroscopy portal is tensioned, the 2 loops tighten. Caution must be exercised to make certain that these 2 loops tension together or 1 loop may end up longer than the other and create a potential surface mass. To avoid this, a probe should be inserted under the loop, which is tightening first, and this loop is pulled out to tighten the second loop. This balances the pulley action and creates a repair in which the knot is buried behind the anchor in the capsule with nothing left on the surface other than 2 strands of suture, of which 55% (the PDS component) should degrade over 2 months. The optimum method of deploying the OmniSpan is to place the first anchor at the superior peripheral surface of the meniscus and the second anchor in the bucket-handle segment, creating a vertical mattress suture repair.

The Meniscal Cinch (Arthrex, Naples, FL, USA), is the newest Arthrex repair device (**Fig. 5**). While there have not been clearly defined versions of the Cinch, the current version is different from that initially released and represents the incremental improvements in their product line, which characterizes Arthrex's approach to innovation. This device is inserted by a "gun" with a needle barrel. There are 2 separate needles, which advance in turn 2 PEEK anchors connected with No. 0 FiberWire (an UHMWPE core surrounded by a braided polyester sleeve). As with other devices, tensioning should be controlled, and when the excess suture is cut, there is no knot left on the surface.

The Sequent meniscal repair device (ConMed Linvatec, Largo, FL, USA) uses No. 0 Hi-Fi (UHMWPE) suture to from 4 or 7 rigid PEEK anchors (**Fig. 6**). This is an all-inside technique, which allows the surgeon to keep the device continuously inside the joint until the repair is complete. The anchors are placed individually through the meniscus with either a straight or a 15° curved needle and deployed at the extracapsular surface. The suture is tensioned using a combination of a ratchet or "freewheeling" setting to control the suture after each anchor is placed. A single Sequent device can be used to place up to 7 anchors. This multianchor design allows for numerous suture configurations from a continuous running stitch to multiple interrupted stitches. The technique is more complex than that associated with other all-inside suture-based devices. This is because in order to lock the suture at each

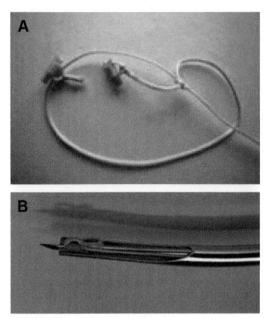

Fig. 5. The Meniscal Cinch *(A)* is inserted by a "gun" *(B)* with a needle barrel. There are 2 separate needles, which advance in turn 2 PEEK anchors connected with No. 0 FiberWire. (*Courtesy of* F. A. Barber MD, Plano, TX.)

anchor a double rotation of the insertion device is required. Also, after the initial PEEK anchor is deployed, subsequent deployments require a cocking of the trigger to advance the next anchor into position before pulling the trigger to deploy the anchor. Once all anchors are placed and sutures tensioned, the suture tail is cut flush with the meniscal surface with a disposable cutter.

The MaxFire MarXmen (Biomet Sports Medicine, Warsaw, IN, USA) is the latest meniscal repair device manufactured by Biomet and is an all-suture implant **(Fig. 7)**. It consists of No. 0 MaxBraid PE (UHMWPE) suture with 2 separate anchors composed of sleeves of braided polyester suture. The MarXmen gun uses a needle to inset the MaxBraid PE suture with its 2 polyester anchors (this is the MaxFire device) through the meniscus similar to the other devices. There are both straight and curved needles available and the anchors can be placed in an either horizontal or vertical

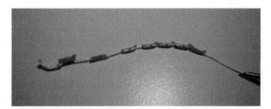

Fig. 6. The Sequent meniscal repair device has a single No. 0 Hi-Fi suture, which spans from four or seven rigid PEEK anchors. The can be inserted one after another to create a continuous running pattern of up to 6 stitches. (*Courtesy of* F. A. Barber MD, Plano, TX.)

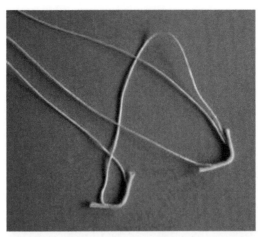

Fig. 7. MarXmen insertion gun inserts the MaxFire repair device. This consists of dual sutures made of No. 0 MaxBraid PE suture. Two short polyester or polyethylene sleeves over this suture serve as anchors when placed through the meniscus. A sliding knot is pushed down the suture to lock the repair in place. (*Courtesy of* F. A. Barber MD, Plano, TX.)

mattress fashion. The sliding, self-locking knot is activated as the suture is tensioned. Also, as with similar designs, once the suture is completely tensioned and the repair secured, the suture tail is cut flush with the meniscus surface.

The CrossFix meniscal repair system (Cayenne Medical, Scottsdale, AZ, USA) is a device that passes a No. 0 Force Fiber (UHMWPE) suture through the meniscus in a horizontal mattress fashion (**Fig. 8**). The device was introduced in 2007 and has 2 parallel, side-by-side 15-gauge needles, either curved 12° or straight, which penetrate the meniscus simultaneously, crossing the tear site. Once the needles have completely penetrated the meniscus, a small shuttling needle passes the suture from one of the side by side needles to the other at the extracapsular portion of the meniscus. As the needles are withdrawn, a 3-mm horizontal mattress stitch is created. As the device is removed completely and the suture tail is pulled, a pre-tied sliding Weston

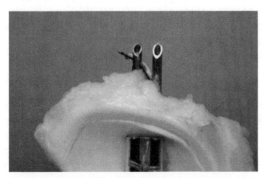

Fig. 8. CrossFix meniscal repair system (Cayenne Medical, Scottsdale, AZ, USA) is a device that passes a No. 0 UHMWPE suture through the meniscus in a horizontal mattress fashion. (*Courtesy of* F. A. Barber MD, Plano, TX.)

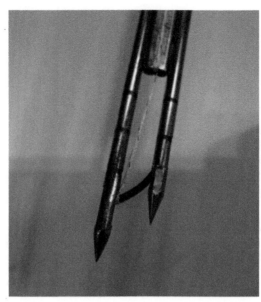

Fig. 9. The Covidien AS (all suture) device has two 15-gauge needles, which are conical in shape and have a polymer coat (NuCoat) to facilitate tissue penetration of No. 2-0 UHMWPE suture. (*Courtesy of* F. A. Barber MD, Plano, TX.)

knot is advanced to the meniscal surface. The meniscus tear is reduced and secured using a knot pusher and standard arthroscopic knot tying techniques can be used to reinforce the Weston knot. The suture ends are then cut at the knot, which sits at the meniscus surface. This device provides an all-arthroscopic, suture-only repair of the meniscus without any implants. Some limitations to the CrossFix include an inability to place sutures in a completely vertical fashion and the prominence of the knot that sits on the meniscus surface, which offers the potential for chondral damage.

The Covidien AS (all suture) device is very similar to the CrossFix and functions in the same fashion. While the two 15-gauge needles are the same size and have 3 mm of separation between them, (the distance from needle tip to needle tip is 5 mm), they are conical in shape and have a polymer coat (NuCoat) to facilitate tissue penetration (**Fig. 9**). This device passes a stitch of No. 2-0 UHMWPE suture with a similar shuttling needle. Both straight and 15° upward curved needles are provided. Another difference from the CrossFix is the prettied modified (with an extra twist wrap) Tennessee slider knot reinforced with 2 half-hitches to secure the repair.

REHABILITATION

Postoperative rehabilitation programs following meniscus repairs are highly variable and a generally accepted protocol does not exist. Key variables to consider include range of motion, weight-bearing status, and return to pivoting sports. With regard to motion, most surgeons would agree that early knee motion is advantageous. Prolonged immobilization can lead to stiffness, atrophy, and decreased collagen content and impaired healing at the meniscus repair site.[32,33] However, terminal knee flexion is associated with considerable posterior translation of the femoral condyles and can magnify stresses within the meniscus.[34,35] Weight-bearing can help reduce and stabilize a bucket-handle meniscus tear,[22] although tibiofemoral loads with increasing knee flexion cause increasing compressive and shear forces in the posterior horn of the meniscus. These forces in the posterior horn can be increased almost 4 times with weight-bearing flexion to 90°.[34] Therefore, weight-bearing in full extension likely poses less risk to meniscal repairs and may aid with healing. Accelerated rehabilitation programs designed to return patients to pivoting sports earlier have been described.[36–38] These permit early full weight-bearing, unrestricted motion, and no limitations on a return to pivoting sports after the postoperative effusion has resolved and full motion is attained. Results of these accelerated programs have shown quicker return of athletes to their chosen sport without compromised results or deleterious effects.

ACL reconstruction associated with a meniscal repair presents its own challenges. Some may wonder if it is necessary to modify the ACL rehabilitation protocol for the meniscus. At present there is no clinical evidence to support slowing the rehabilitation for the associated meniscal repair. While a single unified ACL rehabilitation protocol is difficult develop due to the different properties of different grafts, when there is an associated meniscal repair, slower is not necessarily better. A confounding variable is that the existing clinical data is principally based upon suture repairs and not the newer self-adjusting suture repair devices. As the newer self-adjusting suture devices are more widely adopted, modifications to a postoperative rehabilitation protocol may be justified. These require clinical judgment of the repair strength and quality of the meniscal tissue. Our current preferred protocol for self-adjusting suture devices consists of immediate range of motion from 0 to 90°, immediate full weight-bearing, early close chain strengthening, maintaining flexibility, and endurance. Flexion is limited to 90° for the first 2 months and a full return to pivoting sports is allowed when there is no effusion, full extension, and flexion to 135° is attained.

RESULTS AND COMPLICATIONS

Clinical outcomes following meniscus repair have been reported for most of the surgical techniques described. Studies with long-term follow-up have reported a 79% healing rate for open meniscus repairs[39] and a 73% healing rate for arthroscopic meniscus repairs.[40] The status of the ACL is a critical factor that affects to the overall success of a meniscus repair. Meniscus repairs in ACL-deficient knees have demonstrated a failure rate of 46%, significantly higher than the 5% failure rate seen in stable knees.[37,39] In addition to this meniscus repairs performed in conjunction with anterior cruciate ligament reconstruction have shown better healing rates than isolated meniscal repairs.[41] Other factors that may affect the success of meniscus repair include tear size, tear location, and length of time from injury to repair. Additionally, meniscus repairs performed using nonabsorbable suture demonstrated better results than those performed with absorbable suture.[42]

The clinical results of meniscus repair using the various all-inside meniscal repair devices have been studied. The results of these devices must be compared to the results obtained from the inside-out and outside-in meniscus repairs, which are considered the gold-standard. The overall success rate of the inside-out repair is approximately 82%,[41] similar to the overall success rate of the outside-in repair at 87%.[29] Several studies have looked at all-inside meniscus repairs performed using Arrows. Early published results indicated success rates close to 90%[43–47]; however, over time the failure rates increased to 28% to 41%.[48–50] In addition to this, patients treated with a meniscal Arrow developed numerous complications such as device breakage, soft-tissue inflammation, joint line tenderness, and especially chondral injury, which can occur at a rate of 29%.[50] More promising results have been demonstrated by Meniscal Screws, with a success rate from 83 to 90%,[50–53] and the

BioStinger, with a success rate from 91 to 95%.[54,55] However, they too have had reported complications including device migration.

Published clinical results for all-inside suture-based meniscal repair devices currently are available only for the earliest designs, such as the RapidLoc and FasT-Fix. Overall the RapidLoc has exhibited favorable success rates ranging from 86 to 91%.[56–59] However, in a prospective study the RapidLoc had a 35% failure rate compared to no failures with the outside-in technique and a 5% failure for inside-out suture repairs.[60] Also, there have been several reports of complications from use of the RapidLoc mainly consisting of chondral injury.[61–63] Studies of the FasT-Fix have shown more consistent and promising results. The reported overall success rates for the FasT-Fix range from 82 to 92%.[59,64–68] Not only has the FasT-Fix demonstrated good clinical results, but also few reported complications and little risk to the articular cartilage. The most recently developed meniscal repair devices have not been available long enough to allow an adequate review of the clinical results with the appropriate follow-up. The complications and success rates of these devices cannot be determined at this time.

SUMMARY

Due to advances in meniscus repair techniques, arthroscopic techniques have almost completely replaced open meniscal repairs. The classic inside-out and outside-in suture techniques still have a role in meniscus repair, especially with tears located in anterior meniscal areas that cannot be adequately addressed by all-inside meniscal repair devices. The initial generation of rigid "all-inside" meniscus-fixation devices exhibited promising results, but the risk of significant complications and declining success rates over time have led to their replacement by the self-adjusting suture-based devices. The recent suture-based meniscal fixators have great utility and are becoming widely accepted.[69] The latest suture-based meniscus fixation devices incorporate several similar characteristics in their design. These characteristics include a suture composed at least in part of high strength ultra-high molecular weight polyethylene, anchors that are placed completely extra-articularly, and the elimination of knots or rigid components left on the meniscal surface. These newer designs allow for flexibility in suture placement permitting either horizontal or vertical orientations and decrease the risk of chondral injury.

REFERENCES

1. Ahmed AM, Burke DL. In-vitro measurement of static pressure distribution in synovial joints, part I: tibial surface of the knee. J Biomech Eng 1983;105:216–25.
2. Kurosawa H, Fukubayashi T, Nakajima H. Load-bearing mode of the knee joint: physical behavior of the knee joint with or without menisci. Clin Orthop Relat Res 1980:283–90.
3. Baratz ME, Fu FH, Mengato R. Meniscal tears: the effect of meniscectomy and of repair on intraarticular contact areas and stress in the human knee. A preliminary report. Am J Sports Med 1986;14:270–5.
4. Shoemaker SC, Markolf KL. The role of the meniscus in the anterior-posterior stability of the loaded anterior cruciate-deficient knee. Effects of partial versus total excision. J Bone Joint Surg Am 1986;68:71–9.
5. Fairbank TJ. Knee joint changes after meniscectomy. J Bone Joint Surg Br 1948;30B: 664–70.
6. Annandale T. An operation for displaced semilunar cartilage. Br Med J 1885;1:779.
7. Henning CE, Lynch MA, Clark JR. Vascularity for healing of meniscus repairs. Arthroscopy 1987;3:13–8.

8. Henning CE, Lynch MA, Yearout KM, et al. Arthroscopic meniscal repair using an exogenous fibrin clot. Clin Orthop Relat Res 1990:64–72.
9. Henning CE. Arthroscopic repair of menisci tears. Orthopedics 1983;6:1130–2.
10. Warren RF. Arthroscopic meniscus repair. Arthroscopy 1985;1:170–2.
11. Morgan CD, Casscells SW. Arthroscopic meniscus repair: a safe approach to the posterior horns. Arthroscopy 1986;2:3–12.
12. Morgan CD. The "all-inside" meniscus repair. Arthroscopy 1991;7:120–5.
13. Arnoczky SP, Warren RF. Microvasculature of the human meniscus. Am J Sports Med 1982;10:90–5.
14. Arnoczky SP, Warren RF. The microvasculature of the meniscus and its response to injury. An experimental study in the dog. Am J Sports Med 1983;11:131–41.
15. Okuda K, Ochi M, Shu N, et al. Meniscal rasping for repair of meniscal tear in the avascular zone. Arthroscopy 1999;15:281–6.
16. Uchio Y, Ochi M, Adachi N, et al. Results of rasping of meniscal tears with and without anterior cruciate ligament injury as evaluated by second-look arthroscopy. Arthroscopy 2003;19:463–9.
17. Zhang Z, Arnold JA, Williams T, et al. Repairs by trephination and suturing of longitudinal injuries in the avascular area of the meniscus in goats. Am J Sports Med 1995;23:35–41.
18. Arnoczky SP, Warren RF, Spivak JM. Meniscal repair using an exogenous fibrin clot. An experimental study in dogs. J Bone Joint Surg Am 1988;70:1209–17.
19. Sgaglione NA. Meniscus repair update: current concepts and new techniques. Orthopedics 2005;28:280–6.
20. Morrison JB. Function of the knee joint in various activities. Biomed Eng 1969;4:573–80.
21. Richards DP, Barber FA, Herbert MA. Meniscal tear biomechanics: loads across meniscal tears in human cadaveric knees. Orthopedics 2008;31:347–50.
22. Richards DP, Barber FA, Herbert MA. Compressive loads in longitudinal lateral meniscus tears: a biomechanical study in porcine knees. Arthroscopy 2005;21:1452–6.
23. Becker R, Brettschneider O, Grobel KH, et al. Distraction forces on repaired bucket-handle lesions in the medial meniscus. Am J Sports Med 2006;34:1941–7.
24. Roeddecker K, Muennich U, Nagelschmidt M. Meniscal healing: a biomechanical study. J Surg Res 1994;56:20–7.
25. Morgan CD, Wojtys EM, Casscells CD, et al. Arthroscopic meniscal repair evaluated by second-look arthroscopy. Am J Sports Med 1991;19:632–7; discussion 7–8.
26. Starke C, Kopf S, Petersen W, et al. Meniscal repair. Arthroscopy 2009;25:1033–44.
27. Rosenberg TD, Scott SM, Coward DB, et al. Arthroscopic meniscal repair evaluated with repeat arthroscopy. Arthroscopy 1986;2:14–20.
28. Rimmer MG, Nawana NS, Keene GC, et al. Failure strengths of different meniscal suturing techniques. Arthroscopy 1995;11:146–50.
29. Rodeo SA. Arthroscopic meniscal repair with use of the outside-in technique. Instr Course Lect 2000;49:195–206.
30. Barber FA, McGarry JE. Meniscal repair techniques. Sports Med Arthrosc 2007;15:199–207.
31. Sgaglione NA, Steadman JR, Shaffer B, et al. Current concepts in meniscus surgery: resection to replacement. Arthroscopy 2003;19 Suppl 1:161–88.
32. Klein L, Player JS, Heiple KG, et al. Isotopic evidence for resorption of soft tissues and bone in immobilized dogs. J Bone Joint Surg Am 1982;64:225–30.
33. Dowdy PA, Miniaci A, Arnoczky SP, et al. The effect of cast immobilization on meniscal healing. An experimental study in the dog. Am J Sports Med 1995;23:721–8.

34. Becker R, Wirz D, Wolf C, et al. Measurement of meniscofemoral contact pressure after repair of bucket-handle tears with biodegradable implants. Arch Orthop Trauma Surg 2005;125:254–60.
35. Johal P, Williams A, Wragg P, et al. Tibiofemoral movement in the living knee. A study of weight bearing and nonweight bearing knee kinematics using "interventional" MRI. J Biomech 2005;38:269–76.
36. Barber FA. Accelerated rehabilitation for meniscus repairs. Arthroscopy 1994;10: 206–10.
37. Barber FA, Click SD. Meniscus repair rehabilitation with concurrent anterior cruciate reconstruction. Arthroscopy 1997;13:433–7.
38. Mariani PP, Santori N, Adriani E, et al. Accelerated rehabilitation after arthroscopic meniscal repair: A clinical and magnetic resonance imaging evaluation. Arthroscopy 1996;12:680–6.
39. DeHaven KE, Lohrer WA, Lovelock JE. Long-term results of open meniscal repair. Am J Sports Med 1995;23:524–30.
40. Eggli S, Wegmuller H, Kosina J, et al. Long-term results of arthroscopic meniscal repair. An analysis of isolated tears. Am J Sports Med 1995;23:715–20.
41. Cannon W, Vittori J. The incidence of healing in an arthroscopic meniscal repairs in anterior cruciate ligament-reconstructed knees versus stable knees. Am J Sports Med 1992;20:176–81.
42. Barrett GR, Richardson K, Ruff CG, et al. The effect of suture type on meniscus repair. A clinical analysis. Am J Knee Surg 1997;10:2–9.
43. Albrecht-Olsen P, Kristensen G, Burgaard P, et al. The arrow versus horizontal suture in arthroscopic meniscus repair. A prospective randomized study with arthroscopic evaluation. Knee Surg Sports Traumatol Arthrosc 1999;7:268–73.
44. Hurel C, Mertens F, Verdonk R. Biofix resorbable meniscus arrow for meniscal ruptures: Results of a 1-year follow-up. Knee Surg Sports Traumatol Arthrosc 2000;8:46–52.
45. Petsche TS, Selesnick H, Rochman A. Arthroscopic meniscus repair with bioabsorbable arrows. Arthroscopy 2002;18:246–53.
46. Gill SS, Diduch DR. Outcomes after meniscal repair using the meniscus arrow in knees undergoing concurrent anterior cruciate ligament reconstruction. Arthroscopy 2002;18:569–77.
47. Spindler KP, McCarty EC, Warren TA, et al. Prospective comparison of arthroscopic medial meniscal repair technique: Inside-out suture versus entirely arthroscopic arrows. Am J Sports Med 2003;31:929–34.
48. Kurzweil PR, Tifford CD, Ignacio EM. Unsatisfactory clinical results of meniscal repair using the meniscus arrow. Arthroscopy 2005;21:905e1–7.
49. Lee GP, Diduch DR. Deteriorating outcomes after meniscal repair using the Meniscus Arrow in knees undergoing concurrent anterior cruciate ligament reconstruction: Increased failure rate with long-term follow-up. Am J Sports Med 2005;33:1138–41.
50. Jarvela S, Sihvonen R, Sirkeoja H, et al. All-inside meniscal repair with bioabsorbable meniscal screws or with bioabsorbable meniscus arrows: A prospective, randomized clinical study with 2-year results. Am J Sports Med 2010;38:2211–7.
51. Bohnsack M, Borner C, Schmolke S, et al. Clinical results of arthroscopic meniscal repair using biodegradable screws. Knee Surg Sports Traumatol Arthrosc 2003;11: 379–83.
52. Tsai AM, McAllister DR, Chow S, et al. Results of meniscal repair using a bioabsorbable screw. Arthroscopy 2004;20:586–90.
53. Frosch KH, Fuchs M, Losch A, et al. Repair of meniscal tears with the absorbable Clearfix screw: Results after 1–3 years. Arch Orthop Trauma Surg 2005;125:585–91.

54. Barber FA, Johnson DH, Halbrecht JL. Arthroscopic meniscal repair using the BioStinger. Arthroscopy 2005;21:744–50.
55. Barber FA, Coons DA. Midterm results of meniscal repair using the BioStinger meniscal repair device. Arthroscopy 2006;22:400–5.
56. Quinby JS, Golish SR, Hart JA, et al. All-inside meniscal repair using a new flexible, tensionable device. Am J Sports Med 2006;34:1281–6.
57. Billante MJ, Diduch DR, Lunardini DJ, et al. Meniscal repair using an all-inside, rapidly absorbing, tensionable device. Arthroscopy 2008;24:779–85.
58. Barber FA, Coons DA, Ruiz-Suarez M. Meniscal repair with the RapidLoc meniscal repair device. Arthroscopy 2006;22:962–6.
59. Kalliakmanis A, Zourntos S, Bousgas D, et al. Comparison of arthroscopic meniscal repair results using 3 different meniscal repair devices in anterior cruciate ligament reconstruction patients. Arthroscopy 2008;24:810–6.
60. Hantes ME, Zachos VC, Varitimidis SE, et al. Arthroscopic meniscal repair: A comparative study between three different surgical techniques. Knee Surg Sports Traumatol Arthrosc 2006;14:1232–7.
61. Cohen SB, Anderson MW, Miller MD. Chondral injury after arthroscopic meniscal repair using bioabsorbable Mitek RapidLoc meniscal fixation. Arthroscopy 2003;19: E24–6.
62. Gliatis J, Kouzelis A, Panagopoulos A, et al. Chondral injury due to migration of a Mitek RapidLoc meniscal repair implant after successful meniscal repair: A case report. Knee Surg Sports Traumatol Arthrosc 2005;13:280–2.
63. Barber FA. Chondral injury after meniscal repair with RapidLoc. J Knee Surg 2005; 18:285–8.
64. Haas AL, Schepsis AA, Hornstein J, et al. Meniscal repair using the FasT-Fix all-inside meniscal repair device. Arthroscopy 2005;21:167–75.
65. Kotsovolos ES, Hantes ME, Mastrokalos DS, et al. Results of all-inside meniscal repair with the FasT-Fix meniscal repair system. Arthroscopy 2006;22:3–9.
66. Pujol N, Panarella L, Selmi TAS, et al. Meniscal healing after meniscal repair: A CT arthrography assessment. Am J Sports Med 2008;36:1489–95.
67. Barber FA, Schroeder FA, Oro FB, et al. FasT-Fix meniscal repair: Mid-term results. Arthroscopy 2008;24:1342–8.
68. Tachibana Y, Sakaguchi K, Goto T, et al. Repair integrity evaluated by second-look arthroscopy after arthroscopic meniscal repair with the FasT-Fix during anterior cruciate ligament reconstruction. Am J Sports Med 2010;38:965–1.
69. Redfern J, Burks R. 2009 Survey results: Surgeon practice patterns regarding arthroscopic surgery. Arthroscopy 2009;25:1447–52.

Management of Meniscus Tears that Extend into the Avascular Region

Frank R. Noyes, MD, Sue D. Barber-Westin, BS*

KEYWORDS
- Meniscus tear • Meniscus repair • Avascular region
- Healing • Rehabilitation

The value of the menisci for normal function of the knee joint is well documented. The menisci act as a spacer between the femoral condyle and tibial plateau and limit contact between the articular surfaces. They provide shock absorption to the knee joint during walking and assist in overall lubrication of the articular surfaces.[1,2] The menisci act as a restraint to anteroposterior tibial translation in anterior cruciate ligament (ACL)–deficient knees.[3–5] The lateral meniscus appears to be an important restraint to combined anterior tibial translation and rotation, such as during the pivot-shift maneuver.[5] In the intact knee, removal of the medial meniscus leads to significant increases in anterior tibial translation throughout knee motion.[6] The menisci occupy 60% of the contact area between the tibial and femoral cartilage surfaces, and transmit greater than 50% of joint compression forces. Meniscectomy leads to decreased tibiofemoral contact area by approximately 50% and increased contact forces by 2- to 3-fold.[7–9] Removal of 15% to 34% of a meniscus increases contact pressures by more than 350%.[10] Total lateral meniscectomy results in a 45% to 50% decrease in total contact area and a 235% to 335% increase in peak local contact pressure.[11]

Meniscectomy often results in noteworthy damage to the knee joint, including deterioration and flattening of the articular cartilage surfaces and subchondral bone sclerosis. Removal of the medial meniscus in the intact knee was recently shown in an in vitro model simulation system to elevate friction and cause immediate surface fibrillation, biomechanical wear, and permanent deformation of articular cartilage.[12] Unacceptable long-term clinical results after partial and total meniscectomy have been reported by many investigations.[13–19] Meniscus tears are frequently accompanied by other knee joint injuries. For instance, 40% to 60% of patients who tear the ACL also sustain meniscus tears.[20,21]

The authors have nothing to disclose.
Cincinnati Sportsmedicine Research and Education Foundation, 10663 Montgomery Road, Cincinnati, OH 45242, USA
* Corresponding author.
E-mail address: sbwestin@csmref.org

Preservation of meniscal tissue and function is critical for long-term joint function, especially in younger patients who are athletically active and individuals with strenuous occupations. Early investigations of meniscus repair that focused on simple longitudinal tears located in the periphery or outer one-third region reported high success rates. More recently, several studies have demonstrated satisfactory outcome of repair of complex multiplanar tears that extend into the central third avascular region, leading to justification of the procedure in correctly indicated patients.[22] Two suture techniques exist for meniscus repair. The inside-out technique is preferred because it uses a posteromedial or posterolateral incision and multiple sutures that attach the meniscus directly to its rim with high fixation strength. The all-inside repair technique uses few sutures and has weaker fixation, resulting in the potential of separation at the meniscus repair site and a higher incidence of failure.

CLINICAL EVALUATION

A thorough history is taken that includes assessment of the mechanism of injury, initial and residual symptoms, and current functional limitations. Patients complete questionnaires and are interviewed to rate symptoms, functional limitations, sports and occupational activity levels, and patient perception of the overall knee condition according to the validated Cincinnati Knee Rating System.[23]

A comprehensive examination is conducted to assess gait, range of motion, tibiofemoral pain and crepitus, muscle strength, and ligament stability. Tibiofemoral joint line tenderness is the primary indicator of a meniscus tear. Other clinical signs include pain on forced flexion, lack of full extension, a positive McMurray test, and meniscal displacement during joint compression indicated by popping, clicking, or catching. There may be tenderness on palpation at the posterolateral aspect of the joint at the anatomic site of the popliteomeniscal attachments. The McMurray test is performed in maximum flexion, progressing from maximum external rotation to internal rotation, and then back to external rotation.

Radiographs that are obtained include a lateral at 30° of flexion, patellofemoral axial, and weight-bearing posteroanterior at 45°. Full-standing hip-knee-ankle weight-bearing radiographs are obtained if required to measure varus or valgus malalignment. Magnetic resonance imaging (MRI) using a proton density–weighted, high-resolution, fast-spin-echo sequence is useful to determine the status of the articular cartilage and menisci. MRI has high sensitivity and specificity rates (94% and 81%, respectively) in predicting reparability of longitudinal full-thickness meniscus tears.[24]

CLASSIFICATION OF MENISCUS TEARS

Meniscus tears are classified at arthroscopy according to location, type, and integrity of the tissue.[22] The meniscus is divided into anterior, middle, and posterior thirds as well as inner, middle, and outer thirds. Tears located at the peripheral attachment sites (meniscofemoral and meniscotibial) are referred to as outer third, or red-red tears. Tears located in the middle third are either red-white or white-white. Red-white tears occur at the junction of the outer and middle third regions, approximately 4 mm from the meniscal attachment, with vascular supply present only in the outer third of the tear. White-white tears are located in the inner third region where no blood supply exists.

Single meniscus tears that occur in one plane are classified based on their configuration, such as horizontal, radial, or longitudinal. Complex meniscus tears contain components in multiple planes, including the vertical plane (double or triple longitudinal), vertical and horizontal planes, and vertical and radial planes (flap tears).

Box 1
Indications and contraindications for meniscus repair

Indications

Meniscus tear with tibiofemoral joint line pain

Active patient less than 60 years of age

Concurrent knee ligament reconstruction or osteotomy

Meniscus tear reducible, good tissue integrity, normal position in the joint once repaired

Peripheral single longitudinal tears: red-red, one plane

Middle one-third region: red-white (vascular supply present)

Outer-third and middle-third regions longitudinal, radial, horizontal tears: red-white, one plane: often repairable

Outer-third and middle-third regions complex double or triple longitudinal, flap tears: red-white, multiple planes: repair or excise, see text

Contraindications

Meniscus tears located in inner one-third, white-white region

Chronic degenerative tears in which the tissue is of poor quality, not amendable to suture repair

Longitudinal tears less than 10 mm in length

Incomplete radial tears that do not extend into the outer one-third region

Patient over 60 years of age or sedentary (except traumatic red-red tear to save meniscus)

Patient unwilling to follow postoperative rehabilitation program

Data from Noyes FR, Barber-Westin SD: Meniscus tears: diagnosis, repair techniques, and clinical outcomes. In Noyes' Knee Disorders: Surgery, Rehabilitation, Clinical Outcomes, Saunders, Philadelphia, 2009, pp. 733–71.

INDICATIONS AND CONTRAINDICATIONS FOR MENISCUS REPAIR

The indications and contraindications for meniscus repair are shown in **Box 1** and have been described elsewhere.[22,25] Active patients who are typically in their second to fourth decade of life are excellent candidates. Unstable red-white tears > 10 mm in length in the central third region are often repairable. The meniscus tissue should appear nearly normal, without secondary tears or fragmentation. The tear must be reducible at the time of arthroscopy, with adequate tear site apposition. Patients must agree to comply with the postoperative rehabilitation program and avoid strenuous activities and deep knee flexion for 4 to 6 months.

Meniscus tears in older, sedentary patients or in those unwilling to comply with postoperative rehabilitation are treated with partial resection. Inner third white-white tears are usually excised. Central third white-white tears are only repaired when there is extension into this region from a red-red or red-white tear (such as a large flap tear). Repair is not performed for chronic degenerative tears or stable longitudinal tears < 10 mm in length.

OPERATIVE TECHNIQUES

Complications and results that worsen over time have been reported for all-inside meniscus fixation devices.[26–29] Several studies have analyzed the biomechanical

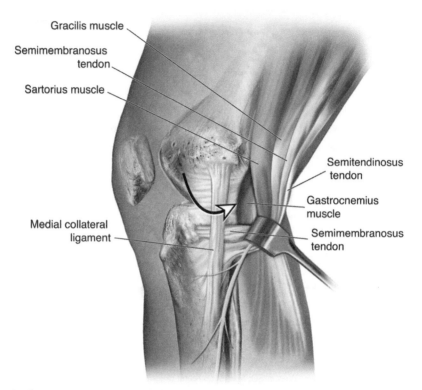

Gracilis muscle

Semimembranosus tendon

Sartorius muscle

Semitendinosus tendon

Gastrocnemius muscle

Medial collateral ligament

Semimembranosus tendon

Fig. 1. The accessory posteromedial approach is shown for a medial meniscus repair. The interval is opened between the posteromedial capsule and the gastrocnemius tendon, just proximal to the semimembranosus tendon (*arrow*). The fascia over the semimembranosus tendon is excised to its tibial attachment to facilitate retrieval of the posterior meniscus sutures. (*Reprinted from* Noyes FR, Barber-Westin SD. Meniscus tears: diagnosis, repair techniques, and clinical outcomes. In: Noyes FR, Barber-Westin SD, editors. Noyes knee disorders: surgery, rehabilitation, clinical outcomes. Philadelphia: Saunders; 2009. p. 733–71; with permission.)

properties of suture techniques and these devices.[30–33] Vertical sutures are superior to both horizontal sutures and meniscus arrows in mean load-to-failure values.[34–36] The superior strength of vertical sutures is believed to be due to the perpendicular orientation to the circumferential collagen bundles of the meniscus.[36] We advocate an inside-out technique using multiple vertical divergent sutures to repair large, unstable meniscus tears that extend into the avascular region.[22]

Diagnostic arthroscopy is first performed and the meniscus tear classified. The meniscus tissue and synovial junction are rasped to stimulate bleeding at the meniscus-synovial border. Loose, unstable meniscus fragments are removed. An accessory 3-cm posteromedial (**Fig. 1**) or posterolateral (**Fig. 2**) exposure is required to protect the neurovascular structures during suture retrieval and knot tying. A popliteal retractor is also used to protect the popliteal neurovascular structures (**Fig. 3**).

The 30° arthroscope is placed through the anteromedial portal for medial meniscus repairs and the anterolateral portal for lateral meniscus repairs for tears located in the posterior third. A single barrel curved or straight cannula is placed in the opposite

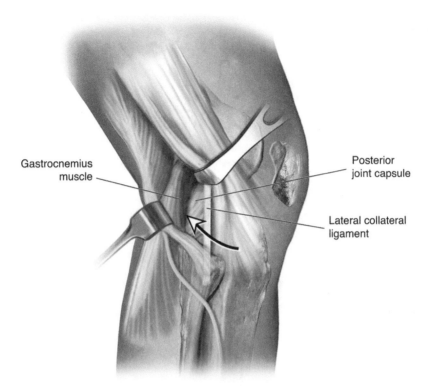

Gastrocnemius
muscle

Posterior
joint capsule

Lateral collateral
ligament

Fig. 2. The accessory posterolateral approach is shown for a lateral meniscus repair. The interval between the lateral gastrocnemius and posterolateral capsule is opened bluntly, just proximal to the fibular head avoiding entering the joint capsule. (*Reprinted from* Noyes FR, Barber-Westin SD. Meniscus tears: diagnosis, repair techniques, and clinical outcomes. In: Noyes FR, Barber-Westin SD, editors. Noyes knee disorders: surgery, rehabilitation, clinical outcomes. Philadelphia: Saunders; 2009. p. 733–71; with permission.)

portal for suture advancement. Curved cannulae are used to direct suture needles away from the midline neurovascular structures. The first vertical sutures are placed at the superior border of the meniscus tear to reduce the meniscus and prevent superior migration when inferior sutures are placed. After anatomic reduction of tear edges, multiple vertical divergent sutures are advanced, retrieved through the accessory posterior incision, and tied directly to the posterior capsule. Sutures are placed every 3 to 5 mm along the tear edges. The close interval between sutures is required to maintain tear site reduction during the prolonged healing time of these avascular repairs.

A double-stacked technique is used for single longitudinal tears (**Fig. 4**). Superior (femoral surface) sutures are placed first to reduce the meniscus to its bed and inferior (tibial surface) sutures are then placed to approximate the inferior portion of the tear (**Fig. 5**). This same technique is used for double longitudinal tears in which the outer tear is near the meniscocapsular junction and the inner tear is near the red-white junction (**Fig. 6**). The peripheral tear is repaired first, followed by the central tear, which is repaired with vertical divergent sutures that span both tear sites (**Fig. 7**).

Radial tears are repaired with horizontal sutures placed at 2- to 4-mm intervals along the tear site (**Fig. 8**). The inner sutures are placed first and securely tied,

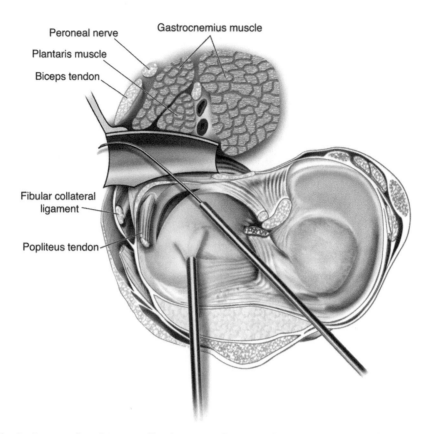

Fig. 3. Cross-section shows popliteal retractor between the lateral gastrocnemius and the posterior capsule. A curved suture cannula is also used to angle the needles away from the neurovascular structures. (*Reprinted from* Noyes FR, Barber-Westin SD. Meniscus tears: diagnosis, repair techniques, and clinical outcomes. In: Noyes FR, Barber-Westin SD, editors. Noyes knee disorders: surgery, rehabilitation, clinical outcomes. Philadelphia: Saunders; 2009. p. 733–71; with permission.)

followed by sutures in the periphery. Three to 4 sutures are used on the superior surface and 1 or 2 sutures are used on the inferior surface. Repair of a flap tear is indicated when the tear extends to the red-white junction or the periphery. Flap tears require 2 sets of sutures (**Fig. 9**). Tension sutures are inserted first through the flap and then into the intact meniscal rim to anchor and reduce the flap into its anatomic bed. With the meniscus reduced, the remaining tear is repaired in the same fashion as a longitudinal tear, with superior and inferior vertical divergent sutures.

STRATEGIES TO AUGMENT HEALING OF MENISCUS REPAIRS

Because avascular meniscus tears do not heal spontaneously,[37–39] a variety of techniques have been attempted to promote a healing response in the treatment of these injuries. Initial techniques used a fibrin clot or trephination to supply growth factors to promote chemotaxis, cell proliferation, and matrix synthesis to the tear site.[39–41] Scott and colleagues[42] reported an increased rate of healing when arthroscopic meniscus repair was combined with dissection of the perimeniscal

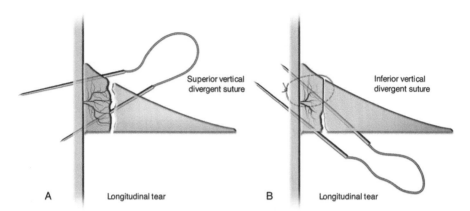

Fig. 4. Double-stacked vertical suture pattern used in the repair of longitudinal meniscus tears. (A) The superior sutures are placed first to close the superior gap and to reduce the meniscus to its bed. (B) Then the inferior suture is placed through the tear to close the inferior gap. (*Reprinted from* Noyes FR, Barber-Westin SD. Meniscus tears: diagnosis, repair techniques, and clinical outcomes. In: Noyes FR, Barber-Westin SD, editors. Noyes knee disorders: surgery, rehabilitation, clinical outcomes. Philadelphia: Saunders; 2009. p. 733–71; with permission.)

synovial membrane. Rasping of the synovium is believed to promote an injury response to assist healing. Early experimental studies reported that synovial cells migrated to the site of avascular meniscus tears[37,43] and resulted in superior healing compared with a fibrin clot.[41] Ochi and colleagues[44] demonstrated that meniscal surface rasping induced cytokines and growth factors that could facilitate meniscal healing.

Cell-based therapy involves transferring tissue-engineered cells seeded onto scaffolds to augment healing of avascular tears.[45–48] In one experimental study,[46] implanting autologous articular chondrocytes onto allogenic meniscal scaffolds with meniscus repair resulted in healing in all specimens. In another experimental study,[47] autologous and allogenic chondrocytes seeded onto a bioabsorbable mesh promoted complete or partial healing of all avascular meniscal lesions. Zellner and colleagues[49] found that precultured chondrogenic mesenchymal stem cells provided enhanced healing of meniscus defects in the avascular region in a rabbit model. Mesenchymal stem cells are attractive because of the potentially unlimited supply and ability to differentiate into specific therapeutic cell types.[50,51] Steinart and colleagues[51] genetically modified bovine meniscal and mesenchymal stem cells to produce transforming growth factor-β1. The cells were inserted with a scaffold into explanted avascular meniscal repair sites. Both cell types resulted in cell proliferation, increased synthesis of proteoglycan and collagen, and histologic healing.

Growth factors hold promise for enhanced healing of avascular tears because they promote cell maturation, differentiation, and proliferation.[52] In an experimental model, meniscal fibrochondrocytes from the avascular region responded to β-fibroblast growth factor by proliferating and creating new extracellular matrix.[53] DNA formation increased 7-fold and protein synthesis increased 15-fold. Authors have identified transforming growth factor-β1 as most effective in stimulating extracellular matrix production by rabbit meniscal fibrochondrocytes.[54]

Platelet-rich plasma (PRP) has generated interest as a healing adjunct for a variety of orthopaedic injuries, conditions, and operations.[55] PRP contains many growth

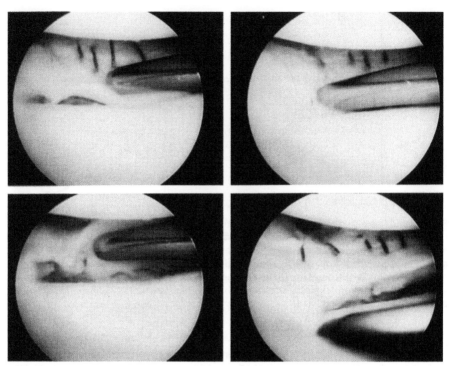

Fig. 5. A longitudinal meniscal tear site demonstrating some fragmentation inferiorly. This tear required multiple superior and inferior vertical divergent sutures to achieve an anatomic reduction. (*Reprinted from* Noyes FR, Barber-Westin SD. Arthroscopic repair of meniscal tears extending into the avascular zone in patients younger than twenty years of age. *Am J Sports Med.* Jul-Aug 2002;30(4):589–600; with permission.)

factors in physiologic proportions that may be advantageous over isolated growth factors. This technique may stimulate chemotaxis, cell proliferation, and angiogenesis. In an experimental study, Ishida and colleagues[56] reported that PRP improved healing based on histology criteria of avascular meniscal defects. In vitro analysis showed enhanced extracellular matrix synthesis and proliferative behavior. However, not all growth factors have been successful in promoting meniscal healing,[57,58] and no clinical study to date has documented their use in meniscus repair. The idea of growth factor or a combination of factors, method of delivery, dosage, and potential side effects require further study.

POSTOPERATIVE REHABILITATION

The rehabilitation program after repair of complex and avascular meniscus tears is summarized in **Table 1**.[59] Immediate knee motion from 0° to 90° is permitted and gradually increased to 0° to 135° by 5 to 6 weeks. Protected, partial weight bearing for 4 to 6 weeks is recommended based on the type of tear. Postoperative signs and symptoms that could indicate a complication and treatment recommendations are summarized in **Table 2**. No squatting or deep flexion activities are permitted for 4 to 6 months, and running, jumping, and cutting are restricted for 6 months to protect the repair site.

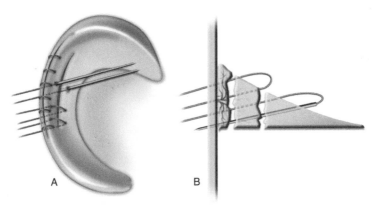

Fig. 6. Double-stacked repair technique for double longitudinal tears. The peripheral tear is stabilized first with superior vertical divergent sutures (*A*), followed by repair of the inner tear in the same fashion (*B*). (*Reprinted from* Noyes FR, Barber-Westin SD. Meniscus tears: diagnosis, repair techniques, and clinical outcomes. In: Noyes FR, Barber-Westin SD, editors. Noyes knee disorders: surgery, rehabilitation, clinical outcomes. Philadelphia: Saunders; 2009. p. 733–71; with permission.)

CLINICAL OUTCOMES OF MENISCUS REPAIR
Authors' Clinical Studies

We have conducted several prospective studies to determine the outcome of inside-out avascular meniscal repair. The first investigation was conducted on 66 patients who underwent a concomitant meniscus repair and ACL reconstruction.[60] All underwent second-look arthroscopy 6 to 25 months postoperatively for symptoms related to either tibial hardware or tibiofemoral joint pain. There were 28 repairs for complex tears that extended into the middle third region. These repairs were

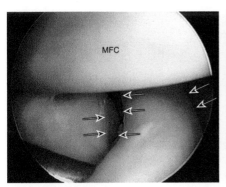
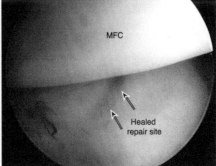

Fig. 7. A double-longitudinal medial meniscus tear with a peripheral tear and another tear at the red-white junction (*left*). Removal of the red-white tear and repair of the peripheral tear would result in substantial loss of meniscus function and accordingly, a repair of both tears was performed. Healing of the tears on subsequent arthroscopy 1 year later (*right*). (*Reprinted from* Noyes FR, Barber-Westin SD. Meniscus tears: diagnosis, repair techniques, and clinical outcomes. In: Noyes FR, Barber-Westin SD, editors. Noyes knee disorders: surgery, rehabilitation, clinical outcomes. Philadelphia: Saunders; 2009. p. 733–71; with permission.)

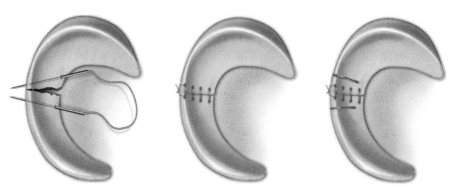

Fig. 8. Repair technique for radial meniscal tears. The inner sutures are placed first, followed by the peripheral sutures. The first suture needle is placed midway through the meniscus body and then used to apply a circumferential tension to reduce the tear gap, then advanced through the posterior meniscus bed. The second suture needle is placed in a similar manner. This reduces the radial gap, allowing subsequent sutures to be placed. Usually, sutures are placed superiorly and 2 sutures, inferiorly. Occasionally, superior vertical divergent sutures are placed along the tear site to help stabilize the repair. (*Reprinted from* Noyes FR, Barber-Westin SD. Meniscus tears: diagnosis, repair techniques, and clinical outcomes. In: Noyes FR, Barber-Westin SD, editors. Noyes knee disorders: surgery, rehabilitation, clinical outcomes. Philadelphia: Saunders; 2009. p. 733–71; with permission.)

classified as completely healed in 54%, partially healed in 32%, and failed in 14%. This early investigation demonstrated an encouraging rate of healing in repair of meniscus tears that extended into the middle third region.

We reported the clinical outcome of 198 meniscus tears that extended into the middle third region or had a rim width of > 4 mm.[61] Patients underwent either a

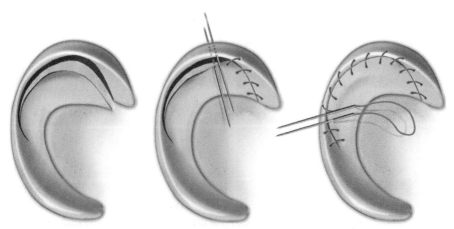

Fig. 9. Repair technique for flap tears. The tear is identified and reduced. Horizontal tension sutures are placed to anchor the radial component of the tear. The longitudinal component is sutured by means of the double-stacked suture technique. (*Reprinted from* Noyes FR, Barber-Westin SD. Meniscus tears: diagnosis, repair techniques, and clinical outcomes. In: Noyes FR, Barber-Westin SD, editors. Noyes knee disorders: surgery, rehabilitation, clinical outcomes. Philadelphia: Saunders; 2009. p. 733–71; with permission.)

Table 1
Rehabilitation protocol summary for repair of meniscus tears extending into the avascular region

	Postoperative Weeks					Postoperative Months			
	1–2	3–4	5–6	7–8	9–12	4	5	6	7–12
Brace: Long-leg postoperative	X	X	X						
Range-of-motion minimum goals									
0°–90°	X								
0°–120°		X							
0°–135°			X						
Weight bearing									
Toe touch: 1/4 body weight	X								
1/2 to 3/4 body weight		X							
Full			X						
Patella mobilization	X	X	X						
Stretching									
Hamstring, gastroc-soleus, iliotibial band, quadriceps	X	X	X	X	X	X	X	X	X
Strengthening									
Quadriceps isometrics, straight leg raises, active knee extension	X	X	X	X	X	X	X	X	X
Closed-chain: gait retraining, toe raises, wall sits, mini-squats			X	X	X	X	X	X	
Knee flexion hamstring curls (90°)				X	X	X	X	X	X
Knee extension quadriceps (90°–30°)			X	X	X	X	X	X	X
Hip abduction-adduction, multi-hip			X	X	X	X	X	X	X
Leg press (70°–10°)					X	X	X	X	X
Balance/proprioceptive training									
Weight-shifting, mini-trampoline, BAPS, BBS, plyometrics			X	X	X	X	X	X	X
Conditioning									
Upper body ergometer		X	X	X					
Bike (stationary)				X	X	X	X	X	X
Aquatic program					X	X	X	X	X
Swimming (kicking)					X	X	X	X	X
Walking					X	X	X	X	X
Stair climbing machine					X	X	X	X	X
Ski machine								X	X
ªRunning: straight								X	X
*Cutting: lateral carioca, figure 8s									X
*Full sports									X

Data from Heckmann T, Barber-Westin SD, Noyes FR. Meniscal repair and transplantation: indications, techniques, rehabilitation, and clinical outcome. J Orthop Sports Phys Ther 2006;36:795–814.
Abbreviations: BAPS, Biomechanical Ankle Platform System (Camp, Jackson, MI, USA); BBS, Biodex Balance System (Shirley, NY, USA).
ª Return to running, cutting, and full sports based on multiple criteria. Patients with noteworthy articular cartilage damage are advised to return to light recreational activities only.

Table 2
Postoperative signs and symptoms requiring prompt treatment

Postoperative Sign, Symptom	Treatment Recommendations
Continued pain in the medial or lateral tibiofemoral compartment of the meniscus repair	Physician examination, assess need for re-repair
Tibiofemoral compartment clicking, or a subjective sensation by the patient of "something being loose" within the tibiofemoral joint	Physician examination, assess need for re-repair
Failure to meet knee extension and flexion goals (see text)	Overpressure program, early gentle manipulation under anesthesia if 0°–135° not met by 6 wk postoperatively
Decreased patellar mobility (indicative of early arthrofibrosis)	Aggressive knee flexion, extension overpressure program, or gentle manipulation under anesthesia to regain full ROM and normal patellar mobility
Decrease in voluntary quadriceps contraction and muscle tone, advancing muscle atrophy	Aggressive quadriceps muscle strengthening program, EMS
Persistent joint effusion, joint inflammation	Aspiration, rule out infection, close physician observation

Data from Heckmann T, Barber-Westin SD, Noyes FR. Meniscal repair and transplantation: indications, techniques, rehabilitation, and clinical outcome. J Orthop Sports Phys Ther 2006;36:795–814.
Abbreviations: ROM, Range of knee motion; EMS, electrical muscle stimulation.

clinical examination a minimum of 2 years postoperatively or follow-up arthroscopy. In this cohort, 126 (71%) underwent ACL reconstruction either with the meniscus repair (96 patients) or a mean of 22 weeks after the repair (30 patients). The overall reoperation rate for tibiofemoral symptoms was 20% (39 meniscus tears). All patients who had tibiofemoral pain underwent follow-up arthroscopy. The reoperation rates according to the type of tear are shown in **Table 3** and the effects of 6 factors on the healing rates are shown in **Table 4**. The results of this investigation support the repair of meniscus tears that extend into the middle third region, especially in patients in their third and fourth decade of life, and competitive athletes.

Table 3
Reoperation rates for meniscal repairs due to tibiofemoral joint symptoms

Type of Meniscus Tear	Total Number of Meniscus Tears in Study	Number Requiring Repeat Arthroscopy
Single longitudinal	92	11 (12%)
Double longitudinal	40	11 (28%)
Complex multiplanar	26	7 (27%)
Radial	15	4 (27%)
Horizontal	14	4 (29%)
Flap	9	2 (22%)
Triple longitudinal	2	0
Total	198	39 (20%)

Table 4
Effect of various factors on healing rates of meniscal repairs that had follow-up arthroscopy

Factor	Healed N	Partially Healed N	Failed N
Tibiofemoral compartment of meniscal repair[a]			
Medial (N = 47)	8	15	24
Lateral (N = 44)	15	20	9
Time from meniscus repair to follow-up arthroscopy[b]			
≤12 mo (N = 61)	18	27	16
>12 mo (N = 30)	5	8	17
Timing of ACL reconstruction			
With meniscal repair (N = 39)	12	18	9
After meniscal repair (N = 27)	9	11	7
Presence of tibiofemoral compartment symptoms[c]			
Symptomatic (N = 39)	2	13	24
Asymptomatic (N = 52)	21	22	9
Time from original knee injury to meniscal repair[d]			
≤10 wk (N = 33)	13	10	10
>10 wk (N = 58)	10	25	23
Patient age			
<25 y (N = 44)	13	17	14
≥25 y (N = 47)	10	18	19

[a] Lateral success rate significantly higher than medial, $P = .008$.
[b] Follow-up arthroscopy less than 12 months postoperative success rate significantly higher than greater than 12 months, $P = .02$.
[c] Tibiofemoral symptoms higher failure rate than no symptoms, $P = .0001$.
[d] Less than 10 weeks from injury higher success rate, $P = .06$.

In a third prospective study, we determined the outcome of meniscus tears that extended into the avascular region in patients greater than 40 years of age.[62] Thirty meniscus repairs in 29 patients were followed up either by clinical examination or second-look arthroscopy. ACL reconstruction was performed at the time of the meniscus repair in 21 patients (72%). At follow-up, 26 meniscus repairs (87%) were asymptomatic and had not required further surgery. There was no significant effect of the tibiofemoral compartment of the meniscus repair, chronicity of injury, concomitant ACL reconstruction, or condition of the articular cartilage on the presence of tibiofemoral pain or meniscus resection. This study showed that repair of complex tears in older adults was feasible and that the majority were asymptomatic an average of 3 years postoperatively.

We conducted a fourth prospective study on 71 meniscus repairs that had been performed in 58 patients under the age of 20 years.[63] Fifty-seven meniscal repairs in 47 knees (80%) were performed concurrently with or before an ACL reconstruction. All knees that had ACL reconstruction were skeletally mature. The initial follow-up evaluation at a mean of 51 months postoperatively showed that 53 of 71 meniscal repairs (75%) had no tibiofemoral symptoms and had not required resection.

From this cohort, a subgroup of 29 meniscus repairs for single longitudinal tears that extended into the avascular zone underwent a long-term evaluation.[64] Clinical evaluation was conducted in 19 repairs (mean, 16.8 years postoperatively), MRI was done in 17 (mean, 17.2 years), and weight-bearing posteroanterior radiographs

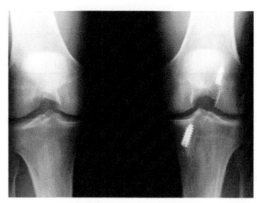

Fig. 10. Standing posteroanterior radiograph 15 years after repair of a 15-mm single longitudinal medial meniscus red-white tear and ACL bone-patellar tendon-bone autograft reconstruction. The 48-year-old man had no symptoms and no decrease in the medial tibiofemoral compartment joint space compared with the contralateral limb. (*Reprinted from* Noyes FR, Barber-Westin SD. Meniscus tears: diagnosis, repair techniques, and clinical outcomes. In: Noyes FR, Barber-Westin SD, editors. Noyes knee disorders: surgery, rehabilitation, clinical outcomes. Philadelphia: Saunders; 2009. p. 733–71; with permission.)

(**Fig. 10**) were obtained in 22 (mean, 16.8 years). The results were determined with 2 validated knee rating systems and assessment of radiographic films and medical records by independent physicians and researchers. A 3 Tesla MRI scanner with cartilage-sensitive pulse sequences, including T2 mapping, was used to study cartilage degeneration and repair site characteristics (**Fig. 11**). Eighteen of the 29 meniscus repairs (62%) were successful, with menisci retained that appeared to be

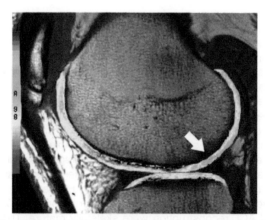

Fig. 11. T2 MRI of a 37-year-old man who is 17 years post-ACL reconstruction and lateral meniscus repair. The patient was asymptomatic with light sports activities. The lateral meniscus repair was healed and the ACL reconstruction restored normal stability. Prolongation of T2 values is noted over the posterior margin with adjacent subchondral sclerosis (*arrow*). (*From* Noyes FR, Chen RC, Barber-Westin SD, et al. Greater than 10-year results of red-white longitudinal meniscus repairs in patients 20 years of age or younger. Am J Sports Med 2011;39:1008–17; with permission.)

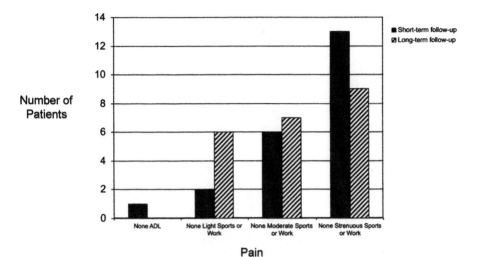

Fig. 12. There was no significant difference in the rating of pain according to activity level between the short-term (mean, 4 years) and long-term (mean, 17 years) follow-up evaluations.

functional. Six repairs required arthroscopic resection, 2 demonstrated loss of joint space on radiographs, and 3 failed according to MRI criteria. There were no significant differences between the short-term (mean, 4 years) and long-term evaluations for the mean scores of pain (**Fig. 12**), swelling, jumping, the patient grade of the overall knee condition (**Fig. 13**), or the overall Cincinnati Knee Rating score.

The results of our investigations allow recommendation of repair of simple or complex meniscal tears that extend into the avascular zone when the appropriate indications are present. This is particularly important in young, active individuals in whom removal of a meniscus tear that extends into the middle avascular region would result in major loss of meniscus function and increased risk for future joint arthrosis. We believe that advanced MRI and weight-bearing posteroanterior radiographs are

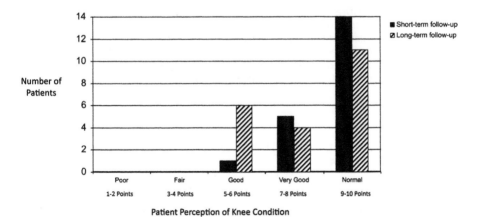

Fig. 13. Patient rating of the overall condition of the knee joint at the short-term (mean, 4 years) and long-term (mean, 17 years) follow-up evaluations.

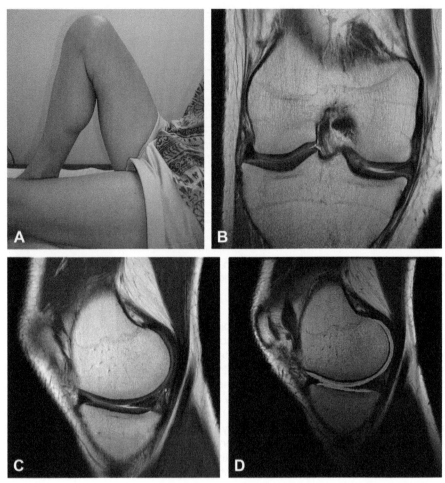

Fig. 14. A 35-year-old woman 20 years after a repair of a 15-mm longitudinal medial meniscus tear involving the posterior horn. The tear extended from the red-white to white-white region, with a 4- to 6-mm meniscus rim. (*A*) The patient is entirely asymptomatic and participates in recreational activities. (*B* and *C*) 3T MRI shows an intact medial meniscus and preserved articular cartilage. (*D*) T2 cartilage mapping shows no focal prolongation of relaxation times. (*Reprinted from* Noyes FR, Barber-Westin SD. Meniscus tears: diagnosis, repair techniques, and clinical outcomes. In: Noyes FR, Barber-Westin SD, editors. Noyes knee disorders: surgery, rehabilitation, clinical outcomes. Philadelphia: Saunders; 2009. p. 733–71; with permission.)

essential to determine the actual failure rate and chondroprotective effects of meniscus repairs (**Fig. 14**).

Outcomes of Other Clinical Studies

A summary of the clinical outcome of meniscal repair from other investigations is shown in **Table 5**.[26–28,65–83] The majority of these studies focused on vertical meniscus suture repair techniques; few reported on the outcome of horizontal suture repair or all-inside

Table 5
Clinical outcome of meniscus repair

Citation	Type Meniscus Tears Number ACL Reconstruction	Surgical Details	Evaluation Methods	Failure Rate	Other Results
Billante et al[65]	N = 38 Red-red: 9 Red-white: 28 White-white: 1 All ACL reconstruction	All-inside, RapidLoc (Depuy Mitek, Raynham, MA, USA) mean, 1.97 devices (range, 1–4)	Physical examination mean, 30.4 mo (range, 21–56)	13%	Failures associated only with gender (males)
Krych et al[67]	N = 47 patients aged ≤ 18 years. Simple, displaced bucket-handle, complex: all isolated	Variety techniques, arrows, inside-out sutures	Physical examination mean, 5.8 y, retrospective chart review	38%	Failures associated with complex tears, rim width ≥ 3 mm
Bryant et al[68]	N = 49 inside-out suture N = 51 arrows All vertical tear in meniscal synovial junction, red-red or red-white zones Prospective, randomized ACL reconstruction in 31 suture group, 34 arrow group	Sutures and arrows placed every 5 mm 10-mm or 13-mm arrows	Physical examination 2 y postop	Suture: 22% Arrow: 21.5%	3 arrows protruded into subcutaneous tissue, one removed. 1 suture required revision. 34 patients could not be randomized because of surgeons' opinions on indications for procedures.
Siebold et al[28]	N = 113 Longitudinal 10–25 mm Red-red or red-white ACL reconstruction: 75	Arrow (Bionex Implants, Blue Bell, PA, USA), 13-mm or 16-mm, mean, 2 (range, 1–4) per repair	Physical examination mean, 6 y (minimum 5 y) postop	28.4%	81.5% failures occurred within 3 years postop

(continued on next page)

Table 5
(continued)

Citation	Type Meniscus Tears Number ACL Reconstruction	Surgical Details	Evaluation Methods	Failure Rate	Other Results
Barber et al[69]	N = 32 All longitudinal, posterior horn Red-red: 11 Red-white: 21 ACL reconstruction: 23	All-inside, RapidLoc mean, 2.2 devices (range, 1–4)	Physical examination mean 31 mo postop (range, 18–48)	12.5%	Chondral grooving observed 1 knee. Surgeon learning curve to avoid cutting suture during device insertion.
Majewski et al[71]	N = 88 Single longitudinal All isolated	Outside-in, 3 to 6 sutures	Physical examination 5 to 17 y postop	24%	8% grade 2/3 x-ray arthrosis involved side compared with grade 0/1 noninvolved side
Kotsovolos et al[72]	N = 61 Longitudinal > 10 mm Red-red: 22 Red-white: 39 ACL reconstruction in 39	All-inside, FasT-Fix (Smith Nephew Endoscopy, Andover, MA, USA), mean, 4.4 anchors	Physical examination 14 to 28 mo postop	9.8%	
Barber and Coons[69]	N = 41 Longitudinal Red-red: 31 Red-white: 10 ACL reconstruction in 35	All-inside, Biostinger (Linvatec, Largo, FL, USA), mean, 2.1 devices (range, 1–4)	Physical examination 24 to 69 mo postop	5%	Device migration 4 knees, 3 repeat surgery. Chondral grooving observed 1 knee.
Quinby et al[66]	N = 54 Red-red: 5 Red-white: 49 All ACL reconstruction	All-inside, RapidLoc mean, 1.8 devices (range, 1–4)	Physical examination mean, 34.8 mo postop (24–50)	9%	
Kurzweil et al[27]	N = 60 Vertical longitudinal, in red-red or red-white zones ACL reconstruction in 45	Arrow	Physical examination 36 to 70 mo postop	28%	20% of failures occurred in knees with ACL reconstruction, normal stability restored. 11% damage femoral articular cartilage 13% of arrows broke during insertion

Study	Tear characteristics	Repair technique	Follow-up	Failure rate	Comments
Haas et al[80]	N = 42 Peripheral longitudinal tears > 10 mm in red-red or red-white zones ACL reconstruction in 22	All-inside, FasT-Fix, mean, 2.8 anchors, vertical, horizontal, or oblique positions used depending on tear	Physical examination 22 to 27 mo postop	12%	Failures associated with bucket-handle tear, multiplanar tears, tears longer than 2 cm, tears > 3 months' duration.
Barber et al[73]	N = 89 Longitudinal, mean 20 mm Red-red: 60 Red-white: 26 White-white: 3 ACL reconstruction in 73	Biostinger: 47 Vertical sutures: 29 Biostinger + sutures: 13	Physical examination 12 to 56 mo postop	Vertical sutures: 0% Biostinger: 8% Biostinger + sutures: 15%	Biostinger unable to repair larger and anteriorly located tears
Kocabey et al[74]	N = 55 Longitudinal, majority 1 to 2 cm Red-red: 29 Red-white: 26 ACL reconstruction in 32	All-inside, T-Fix (Smith Nephew Endoscopy, Andover, MA, USA), 2 to 6 devices used, horizontal mattress suture configuration	Physical examination 4 to 24 mo postop	13%	Rehabilitation program altered depending on type and size of meniscus tear
Steenbrugge et al[75]	N = 45 Red-red: 15 Red-white: 28 White-white: 2 ACL torn in 7 in inside-out group, not reconstructed ACL torn in 9 in arrow group, reconstructed in 6	Inside-out: 20, vertical sutures placed 3- to 4-mm intervals All-inside arrow (Biofix, Bioscience, Tampere, Finland): 25, inserted every 5 to 10 mm	Physical examination 6 to 15 y postop	Suture: 0% Arrow: 12%	

(continued on next page)

Table 5
(continued)

Citation	Type Meniscus Tears Number ACL Reconstruction	Surgical Details	Evaluation Methods	Failure Rate	Other Results
Spindler et al[76]	N = 125 medial meniscus tears. In peripheral in majority. ACL reconstructed in all knees	Inside-out: 40, horizontal. All inside arrow: 85	Physical examination 68 mo median suture group 27 mo median arrow group	Suture: 12.5% Arrow: 11%	
O'Shea et al[77]	N = 55 locked bucket handle tears. Red-red: 1. Red-white: 11. White-white: 43. ACL reconstruction staged mean 77 days after meniscus repair	Inside-out, 3 to 6 vertical mattress sutures	Follow-up arthroscopy mean 77 d postop, Physical examination mean 4.3 y postop	Red-red: 0% Red-white: 9% White-white: 19%	
Kurosaka et al[78]	N = 114 chronic vertical or vertical-oblique tear, in periphery > 1 cm in length. ACL reconstruction in 102 of 111 patients (92%)	Inside-out, vertical sutures	Follow-up arthroscopy mean, 13 mo (range, 2–32) Physical examination mean, 54 mo (17–84) after follow-up arthroscopy	32%	Follow-up arthroscopy showed 79% healed. 13 repairs initially healed failed later postoperative.
Rodeo[79]	N = 90. Red-red: 78. Red-white: 10. White-white: 2. ACL reconstruction in 38 patients (42%)	Outside-in, vertical sutures placed every 3 to 4 mm	Physical examination mean, 46 mo (36–89) MRI, CT, or scope in 86	13% Red-white: 40%	Failures correlated with uncorrected ACL deficiency, tears in central third region, tears in posterior horn of medial meniscus

Data from Noyes FR, Barber-Westin SD: Meniscus tears: diganosis, repair techniques, and clinical outcomes. In Noyes' Knee Disorders: Surgery, Rehabilitation, Clinical Outcomes. Noyes FR, Barber-Westin SD (eds.), Saunders, Philadelphia, 2009, pp. 733–71.

fixators. Failure rates vary greatly, along with the effects of the side of meniscus tear, concurrent ACL reconstruction, location of meniscus tear, age, and gender.

Investigations of newer all-inside suture systems have reported acceptable failure rates between 9% and 13%.[65,66,72,80,84] However, longer-term follow-up is required to ensure that the rate of failure of these systems does not increase with time. In addition, we believe that the use of only 2 to 3 sutures, as used with all-inside suture systems, provides inadequate stabilization and is inferior to multiple vertical divergent suture techniques. Complications and deteriorating results have been reported after the early use of all-inside fixation devices.[26–28,84] Lee and Diduch[26] reported an increasing rate of failure with time in 28 patients who underwent meniscus repair with the Meniscus Arrow (Bionx, Blue Bell, PA, USA) and a concomitant ACL reconstruction. The initial success rate of 90.6% reported a mean of 2.3 years postoperatively decreased to 71.4% at 6.6 years.

SUMMARY

The question of whether meniscal repair is effective in providing chondroprotective effects to the knee joint remains unanswered. However, the well-documented irreparable joint damage and poor results of long-term clinical studies after partial and total meniscectomy justify preservation of meniscal tissue whenever possible. We believe that the gold standard operative technique is a meticulous inside-out repair with multiple vertical divergent sutures and an accessory posteromedial or postero-lateral approach to tie the sutures directly posterior to the meniscus attachment. We consider meniscus repair as important, if not more important, as an ACL reconstruction in regard to long-term knee function.

We disagree with the approach of leaving a meniscus tear that is > 10 mm in length untreated at the time of ACL reconstruction, because this may risk future tearing and subsequent loss of meniscus function. Once a meniscectomy has been performed in a young patient, few options exist. It is unfortunate that, in many patients requiring meniscus transplantation, the original treatment of the meniscus tear was ineffective. Either a tear was left untreated that subsequently required resection, a repair was done with too few sutures or with fixators that provided limited stability and failed, or a major tear that extended into the central avascular region was removed, which could have been repaired.

In the future, tissue engineering may increase the success rates of meniscus repair for tears that extend into the avascular region. Cell-based therapy using meniscal fibrochondrocytes or articular chondrocytes or mesenchymal stem cells seeded onto scaffolds offers promise, as does the introduction of growth factors into repair sites.

REFERENCES

1. Voloshin AS, Wosk J. Shock absorption of meniscectomized and painful knees: a comparative in vivo study. J Biomed Eng 1983;5(2):157–61.
2. Mow VC, Ratcliffe A, Chern KY, et al. Structure and function relationships of the menisci of the knee. In: Mow VC, Arnoczky SP, Jackson DW, editors. Knee meniscus: basic and clinical foundations. New York: Raven Press, Ltd.; 1992. p. 37–57.
3. Markolf KL, Mensch JS, Amstutz HC. Stiffness and laxity of the knee—the contributions of the supporting structures. A quantitative in vitro study. J Bone Joint Surg Am 1976;58(5):583–94.
4. Shoemaker SC, Markolf KI. The role of the meniscus in the anterior-posterior stability of the loaded anterior cruciate-deficient knee. Effects of partial versus total excision. J Bone Joint Surg 1986;68A(1):71–9.

5. Musahl V, Citak M, O'Loughlin PF, et al. The effect of medial versus lateral meniscectomy on the stability of the anterior cruciate ligament-deficient knee. Am J Sports Med 2010;38(8):1591–7.
6. Spang JT, Dang AB, Mazzocca A, et al. The effect of medial meniscectomy and meniscal allograft transplantation on knee and anterior cruciate ligament biomechanics. Arthroscopy 2010;26(2):192–201.
7. Ahmed AM, Burke DL. In-vitro measurement of static pressure distribution in synovial joints—part I: tibial surface of the knee. J Biomech Eng 1983;105(3):216–25.
8. Verma NN, Kolb E, Cole BJ, et al. The effects of medial meniscal transplantation techniques on intra-articular contact pressures. J Knee Surg 2008;21(1):20–6.
9. McDermott ID, Lie DT, Edwards A, et al. The effects of lateral meniscal allograft transplantation techniques on tibio-femoral contact pressures. Knee Surg Sports Traumatol Arthrosc 2008;16(6):553–60.
10. Seedhom BB, Hargreaves DJ. Transmission of the load in the knee joint with special reference to the role of the menisci. Part II. Experimental results, discussion, and conclusions. Eng Med 1979;8:220–8.
11. Paletta GA, Manning T, Snell E, et al. The effect of allograft meniscal replacement on intraarticular contact area and pressures in the human knee. A biomechanical study. Am J Sports Med 1997;25(5):692–8.
12. McCann L, Ingham E, Jin Z, et al. Influence of the meniscus on friction and degradation of cartilage in the natural knee joint. Osteoarthr Cartil 2009;17(8): 995–1000.
13. Stein T, Mehling AP, Welsch F, et al. Long-term outcome after arthroscopic meniscal repair versus arthroscopic partial meniscectomy for traumatic meniscal tears. Am J Sports Med 2010;38(8):1542–8.
14. Andersson-Molina H, Karlsson H, Rockborn P. Arthroscopic partial and total meniscectomy: a long-term follow-up study with matched controls. Arthroscopy 2002; 18(2):183–9.
15. Rockborn P, Messner K. Long-term results of meniscus repair and meniscectomy: a 13-year functional and radiographic follow-up study. Knee Surg Sports Traumatol Arthrosc 2000;8(1):2–10.
16. Roos EM, Ostenberg A, Roos H, et al. Long-term outcome of meniscectomy: symptoms, function, and performance tests in patients with or without radiographic osteoarthritis compared to matched controls. Osteoarthr Cartil 2001;9(4): 316–24.
17. Scheller G, Sobau C, Bulow JU. Arthroscopic partial lateral meniscectomy in an otherwise normal knee: clinical, functional, and radiographic results of a long-term follow-up study. Arthroscopy 2001;17(9):946–52.
18. McNicholas MJ, Rowley DI, McGurty D, et al. Total meniscectomy in adolescence. A thirty-year follow-up. J Bone Joint Surg Br 2000;82(2):217–21.
19. Magnussen RA, Mansour AA, Carey JL, et al. Meniscus status at anterior cruciate ligament reconstruction associated with radiographic signs of osteoarthritis at 5- to 10-year follow-up: a systematic review. J Knee Surg 2009;22(4):347–57.
20. Levy AS, Meier SW. Approach to cartilage injury in the anterior cruciate ligament-deficient knee. Orthop Clin North Am 2003;34(1):149–67.
21. Noyes FR, Bassett RW, Grood ES, et al. Arthroscopy in acute traumatic hemarthrosis of the knee. Incidence of anterior cruciate tears and other injuries. J Bone Joint Surg Am 1980;62(5):687–95, 757.
22. Noyes FR, Barber-Westin SD. Meniscus tears: diagnosis, repair techniques, and clinical outcomes. In: Noyes FR, Barber-Westin SD, editors. Noyes knee disorders: surgery, rehabilitation, clinical outcomes. Philadelphia: Saunders; 2009. p. 733–71.

23. Barber-Westin SD, Noyes FR, McCloskey JW. Rigorous statistical reliability, validity, and responsiveness testing of the Cincinnati knee rating system in 350 subjects with uninjured, injured, or anterior cruciate ligament-reconstructed knees. Am J Sports Med 1999;27(4):402–16.

24. Nourissat G, Beaufils P, Charrois O, et al. Magnetic resonance imaging as a tool to predict reparability of longitudinal full-thickness meniscus lesions. Knee Surg Sports Traumatol Arthrosc 2008;16(5):482–6.

25. Noyes FR, Barber-Westin SD. Repair of complex and avascular meniscal tears and meniscal transplantation. J Bone Joint Surg Am 2010;92(4):1012–29.

26. Lee GP, Diduch DR. Deteriorating outcomes after meniscal repair using the meniscus arrow in knees undergoing concurrent anterior cruciate ligament recon-struction: increased failure rate with long-term follow-up. Am J Sports Med 2005;33(8):1138–41.

27. Kurzweil PR, Tifford CD, Ignacio EM. Unsatisfactory clinical results of meniscal repair using the meniscus arrow. Arthroscopy 2005;21(8):905,e901–905.e907.

28. Siebold R, Dehler C, Boes L, et al. Arthroscopic all-inside repair using the Meniscus Arrow: long-term clinical follow-up of 113 patients. Arthroscopy 2007; 23(4):394–9.

29. Lozano J, Ma CB, Cannon WD. All-inside meniscus repair: a systematic review. Clin Orthop Relat Res 2007;455:134–41.

30. Zantop T, Eggers AK, Weimann A, et al. Initial fixation strength of flexible all-inside meniscus suture anchors in comparison to conventional suture technique and rigid anchors: biomechanical evaluation of new meniscus refixation systems. Am J Sports Med 2004;32(4):863–9.

31. Zantop T, Ruemmler M, Welbers B, et al. Cyclic loading comparison between biodegradable interference screw fixation and biodegradable double cross-pin fixation of human bone-patellar tendon-bone grafts. Arthroscopy 2005;21(8): 934–41.

32. Barber FA, Herbert MA, Richards DP. Load to failure testing of new meniscal repair devices. Arthroscopy 2004;20(1):45–50.

33. Miller MD, Kline AJ, Jepsen KG. "All-inside" meniscal repair devices: an experimental study in the goat model. Am J Sports Med 2004;32(4):858–62.

34. Farng E, Sherman O. Meniscal repair devices: a clinical and biomechanical literature review. Arthroscopy 2004;20(3):273–86.

35. Asik M, Sener N. Failure strength of repair devices versus meniscus suturing tech-niques. Knee Surg Sports Traumatol Arthrosc 2002;10(1):25–9.

36. Rankin CC, Lintner DM, Noble PC, et al. A biomechanical analysis of meniscal repair techniques. Am J Sports Med 2002;30(4):492–7.

37. Arnoczky SP, Warren RF. The microvasculature of the meniscus and its response to injury. An experimental study in the dog. Am J Sports Med 1983;11:131–41.

38. Zhang ZN, Tu KY, Xu YK, et al. Treatment of longitudinal injuries in avascular area of meniscus in dogs by trephination. Arthroscopy 1988;4(3):151–9.

39. Port J, Jackson DW, Lee TQ, et al. Meniscal repair supplemented with exogenous fibrin clot and autogenous cultured marrow cells in the goat model. Am J Sports Med 1996;24(4):547–55.

40. Arnoczky SP, Warren RF, Spivak JM. Meniscal repair using an exogenous fibrin clot. An experimental study in dogs. J Bone Joint Surg 1988;70A(8):1209–17.

41. Ritchie JR, Miller MD, Bents RT, et al. Meniscal repair in the goat model. The use of healing adjuncts on central tears and the role of magnetic resonance arthrography in repair evaluation. Am J Sports Med 1998;26(2):278–84.

42. Scott GA, Jolly BL, Henning CE. Combined posterior incision and arthroscopic intra-articular repair of the meniscus: an examination of factors affecting healing. J Bone Joint Surg 1986;68A(6):847–61.

43. Okuda K, Ochi M, Shu N, et al. Meniscal rasping for repair of meniscal tear in the avascular zone. Arthroscopy 1999;15(3):281–6.

44. Ochi M, Uchio Y, Okuda K, et al. Expression of cytokines after meniscal rasping to promote meniscal healing. Arthroscopy 2001;17(7):724–31.

45. Pabbruwe MB, Kafienah W, Tarlton JF, et al. Repair of meniscal cartilage white zone tears using a stem cell/collagen-scaffold implant. Biomaterials 2010;31(9):2583–91.

46. Peretti GM, Gill TJ, Xu JW, et al. Cell-based therapy for meniscal repair: a large animal study. Am J Sports Med 2004;32(1):146–58.

47. Weinand C, Peretti GM, Adams SB, Jr, et al. An allogenic cell-based implant for meniscal lesions. Am J Sports Med 2006;34(11):1779–89.

48. Fox DB, Warnock JJ, Stoker AM, et al. Effects of growth factors on equine synovial fibroblasts seeded on synthetic scaffolds for avascular meniscal tissue engineering. Res Vet Sci 2010;88(2):326–32.

49. Zellner J, Mueller M, Berner A, et al. Role of mesenchymal stem cells in tissue engineering of meniscus. J Biomed Mater Res A 2010;94(4):1150–61.

50. Izuta Y, Ochi M, Adachi N, et al. Meniscal repair using bone marrow-derived mesenchymal stem cells: experimental study using green fluorescent protein transgenic rats. Knee 2005;12(3):217–23.

51. Steinert AF, Palmer GD, Capito R, et al. Genetically enhanced engineering of meniscus tissue using ex vivo delivery of transforming growth factor-beta 1 complementary deoxyribonucleic acid. Tissue Eng 2007;13(9):2227–37.

52. Forriol F. Growth factors in cartilage and meniscus repair. Injury 2009;40(Suppl 3): S12–6.

53. Tumia NS, Johnstone AJ. Promoting the proliferative and synthetic activity of knee meniscal fibrochondrocytes using basic fibroblast growth factor in vitro. Am J Sports Med 2004;32(4):915–20.

54. Pangborn CA, Athanasiou KA. Growth factors and fibrochondrocytes in scaffolds. J Orthop Res 2005;23(5):1184–90.

55. Foster TE, Puskas BL, Mandelbaum BR, et al. Platelet-rich plasma: from basic science to clinical applications. Am J Sports Med 2009;37(11):2259–72.

56. Ishida K, Kuroda R, Miwa M, et al. The regenerative effects of platelet-rich plasma on meniscal cells in vitro and its in vivo application with biodegradable gelatin hydrogel. Tissue Eng 2007;13(5):1103–12.

57. Petersen W, Pufe T, Starke C, et al. The effect of locally applied vascular endothelial growth factor on meniscus healing: gross and histological findings. Arch Orthop Trauma Surg 2007;127(4):235–40.

58. Spindler KP, Mayes CE, Miller RR, et al. Regional mitogenic response of the meniscus to platelet-derived growth factor (PDGF-AB). J Orthop Res 1995;13(2):201–7.

59. Heckmann TP, Noyes FR, Barber-Westin SD. Rehabilitation of meniscus repair and transplantation procedures. In: Noyes FR, Barber-Westin SD, editors. Noyes knee disorders: surgery, rehabilitation, clinical outcomes. Philadelphia: Saunders; 2009. p. 806–17.

60. Buseck MS, Noyes FR. Arthroscopic evaluation of meniscal repairs after anterior cruciate ligament reconstruction and immediate motion. Am J Sports Med 1991; 19(5):489–94.

61. Rubman MH, Noyes FR, Barber-Westin SD. Arthroscopic repair of meniscal tears that extend into the avascular zone. A review of 198 single and complex tears. Am J Sports Med 1998;26(1):87–95.

62. Noyes FR, Barber-Westin SD. Arthroscopic repair of meniscus tears extending into the avascular zone with or without anterior cruciate ligament reconstruction in patients 40 years of age and older. Arthroscopy 2000;16(8):822–9.

63. Noyes FR, Barber-Westin SD. Arthroscopic repair of meniscal tears extending into the avascular zone in patients younger than twenty years of age. Am J Sports Med 2002;30(4):589–600.

64. Noyes FR, Chen RC, Barber-Westin SD, et al. Greater than 10-year results of red-white longitudinal meniscus repairs in patients 20 years of age or younger. Am J Sports Med 2011;39(5):1008–17.

65. Billante MJ, Diduch DR, Lunardini DJ, et al. Meniscal repair using an all-inside, rapidly absorbing, tensionable device. Arthroscopy 2008;24(7):779–85.

66. Quinby JS, Golish SR, Hart JA, et al. All-inside meniscal repair using a new flexible, tensionable device. Am J Sports Med 2006;34(8):1281–6.

67. Krych AJ, McIntosh AL, Voll AE, et al. Arthroscopic repair of isolated meniscal tears in patients 18 years and younger. Am J Sports Med 2008;36(7):1283–9.

68. Bryant D, Dill J, Litchfield R, et al. Effectiveness of bioabsorbable arrows compared with inside-out suturing for vertical, reparable meniscal lesions: a randomized clinical trial. Am J Sports Med 2007;35(6):889–96.

69. Barber FA, Coons DA, Ruiz-Suarez M. Meniscal repair with the RapidLoc meniscal repair device. Arthroscopy 2006;22(9):962–6.

70. Barber FA, Coons DA. Midterm results of meniscal repair using the BioStinger meniscal repair device. Arthroscopy 2006;22(4):400–5.

71. Majewski M, Stoll R, Widmer H, et al. Midterm and long-term results after arthroscopic suture repair of isolated, longitudinal, vertical meniscal tears in stable knees. Am J Sports Med 2006;34(7):1072–6.

72. Kotsovolos ES, Hantes ME, Mastrokalos DS. Results of all-inside meniscal repair with the FasT-Fix meniscal repair system. Arthroscopy 2006;22(1):3–9.

73. Barber FA, Johnson DH, Halbrecht JL. Arthroscopic meniscal repair using the BioStinger. Arthroscopy 2005;21(6):744–50.

74. Kocabey Y, Nyland J, Isbell WM, et al. Patient outcomes following T-Fix meniscal repair and a modifiable, progressive rehabilitation program, a retrospective study. Arch Orthop Trauma Surg 2004;124(9):592–6.

75. Steenbrugge F, Verdonk R, Hurel C, et al. Arthroscopic meniscus repair: inside-out technique vs. Biofix meniscus arrow. Knee Surg Sports Traumatol Arthrosc 2004; 12(1):43–9.

76. Spindler KP, McCarty EC, Warren TA, et al. Prospective comparison of arthroscopic medial meniscal repair technique: inside-out suture versus entirely arthroscopic arrows. Am J Sports Med 2003;31(6):929–34.

77. O'Shea JJ, Shelbourne KD. Repair of locked bucket-handle meniscal tears in knees with chronic anterior cruciate ligament deficiency. Am J Sports Med 2003;31(2):216–20.

78. Kurosaka M, Yoshiya S, Kuroda R, et al. Repeat tears of repaired menisci after arthroscopic confirmation of healing. J Bone Joint Surg Br 2002;84(1):34–7.

79. Rodeo SA. Arthroscopic meniscal repair with use of the outside-in technique. J Bone Joint Surg Am 2000;82-A(1):127–41.

80. Haas AL, Schepsis AA, Hornstein J, et al. Meniscal repair using the FasT-Fix all-inside meniscal repair device. Arthroscopy 2005;21(2):167–75.

81. Horibe S, Shino K, Maeda A, et al. Results of isolated meniscal repair evaluated by second-look arthroscopy. Arthroscopy 1996;12(2):150–5.

82. DeHaven KE, Lohrer WA, Lovelock JE. Long-term results of open meniscal repair. Am J Sports Med 1995;23(5):524–30.

83. Ellermann A, Siebold R, Buelow JU, et al. Clinical evaluation of meniscus repair with a bioabsorbable arrow: a 2- to 3-year follow-up study. Knee Surg Sports Traumatol Arthrosc 2002;10(5):289–93.

84. Kalliakmanis A, Zourntos S, Bousgas D, et al. Comparison of arthroscopic meniscal repair results using 3 different meniscal repair devices in anterior cruciate ligament reconstruction patients. Arthroscopy 2008;24(7):810–6.

Biologic Enhancement of Meniscus Repair

Laura E. Scordino, MD, Thomas M. DeBerardino, MD*

KEYWORDS

- Platelet-rich plasma • Blood clot • Fibrin clot • Biologic
- Meniscus • Meniscal repair • PRP

The first meniscal repair was described by Annandale in 1885.[1] In addition to the patients' reported 1-month stay in the hospital, many other changes have occurred in the techniques of meniscal repair since that time.[1] Most repairs are performed arthroscopically, with a variety of suture techniques ranging from inside-out, outside-in, to all-inside. Regardless of the technique utilized, vertical suture placement is one of the cornerstones of meniscal repair. Meniscal repair techniques are discussed elsewhere in this *Clinics in Sports Medicine* issue and will not be further discussed herein.

Since the 1980s, biologic enhancement of meniscal repair has been reported. Initially, fibrin clot was used to augment meniscal repairs in avascular zones of injury. Recently, the use of platelet-rich plasma (PRP) to enhance spinal fusions, as well as tendon and ligament repair, has been carried over to studies involving its use in meniscal repair. Furthermore, basic science and animal studies have involved tissue engineering and the local delivery of growth factors in the enhancement of meniscal repair. This article discusses the use of biologic products to enhance meniscal repair.

FUNCTION

Although Annandale described the first meniscal repair in 1885, and Fairbank first described degenerative changes that occurred after meniscectomy in 1948, removal of part or all of the meniscus was the treatment of choice until the 1960s and 1970s.[2,3] Since then, it has been understood that the meniscus plays an important anatomic function in knee kinematics.

One important function of the meniscus is to transmit compressive loads. Biomechanical studies have found that it is responsible for transmitting 50% of body weight load in extension and up to 85% in 90° of flexion.[4,5] Thus, debridement of even part

---

Financial Disclaimer: The senior author is provided funding by an unrestricted educational grant from Arthrex, Inc, Naples, Florida.

Department of Orthopaedics, University of Connecticut, Medical Arts and Research Building, 263 Farmington Avenue, Farmington, CT 06034-4038, USA
* Corresponding author.
E-mail address: tdeber@uchc.edu

of the meniscus can result in decreased contact area, which can then results in increased contact pressures.

Another function of the meniscus is to act as a shock absorber during gate. Biomechanical studies have found that normal knees have a 20% higher shock-absorbing capacity than knees treated with meniscetomy.[6]

Although definitive studies are lacking, it has been suggested that by increasing the congruity between the femoral and tibial condyles, the meniscus helps maintain articular lubrication.[2] Also, type I and type II nerve endings observed in the anterior and posterior horns of the meniscus suggest that it may also play a role in proprioception.[7,8]

ANATOMY

The menisci are semicircular fibrocartilage disks positioned between the femur and the tibia. The medial meniscus is larger than the lateral meniscus in anterior-to-posterior diameter; it is approximately 3.5 cm long. It is thicker posteriorly than anteriorly. The medial meniscus has several points of fixation. Anteriorly, it is attached to the tibia in the intercondylar fossa, just anterior to the footprint of the anterior cruciate ligament. Its posterior insertion point is between the posterior insertion of the lateral collateral ligament and the footprint of the posterior cruciate ligament. Along the periphery, the medial meniscus is strongly attached to tibia through the coronary ligament as well as to a thickening of the medial joint capsule referred to as *the deep medial collateral ligament*.

The lateral meniscus, however, is more circular and covers almost 75% of the articular surface of the more convex lateral tibial plateau. Its anterior insertion point on the tibia is slightly posterior to the footprint of the anterior cruciate ligament. Its posterior insertion point is anterior to the insertion of both the medial meniscus and posterior cruciate ligament. The tibia has strong posterior attachments to the femur, referred to as *the ligament of Humphry*, which runs anterior to the posterior cruciate ligament, as well as the ligament of Wrisberg. Also, the popliteal hiatus is an area unique to the lateral meniscus. This is the area in which the popliteal tendon runs through the knee joint interrupting the lateral meniscus attachment to the joint capsule. This in part contributes to the fact that the lateral meniscus is more mobile than the medial meniscus.[2]

The extracellular matrix of the meniscus is composed of water and collagen, primarily type I collagen (almost 90%), but types II, III, V, and VI had been identified as well, as well as proteogylcan. Collagen fibers are lined up circumferentially along the middle length of the meniscus and act to transmit load across the knee joint. A smaller portion of collagen fibers are lined radially within the substance of the meniscus to potentially resist the longitudinal splitting of the meniscus under compressive forces.[2,9]

VASCULARITY

The vascular supply to the various portions of the meniscus forms the basis of treatment options. The meniscus is a relatively avascular structure. The lateral and medial geniculate arteries give rise to the perimeniscal capillary plexus (PCP). This plexus surrounds the periphery of the meniscus providing blood mostly to the outer third of the meniscus, with the central portion of the meniscus receiving progressively less blood supply. Anatomic studies have shown that this arborization of blood vessels penetrates only approximately 10% to 30% the width of the medial meniscus and 10% to 25% of the lateral meniscus. A vascular synovial membrane covers the area surrounding the femoral and tibial articular attachments of the meniscus.[2,10] As such, meniscal tears have been described based on their location within the meniscus relative to the periphery and thus the vascular supply. Meniscal tears are said to fall within the red-red, or most vascular peripheral third; red-white, or middle third; and white-white, or avascular central third. When considering whether a meniscal tear is repairable, the location of a meniscal tear relative to the periphery is just as, if not more, important than the type of meniscal tear itself.

Of note, in addition to the central portion of the meniscus, the area of the popliteal hiatus in the lateral meniscus has also been described as an avascular area.[2]

HEALING

Understanding how the meniscus naturally heals tears is the key to both the development and the application of biological enhancement of meniscal repairs today. The most important fact to recall is that the basis of vascularity of the meniscus comes from the PCP. When a tear occurs in the peripheral third, a fibrin clot forms, which is rich in inflammatory cells. The PCP grows rapidly over the fibrin conduit, as well as into the fibrous scar, while contributing undifferentiated mesenchymal cells. Studies have found that tears within the vascular peripheral zone are completely healed by a fibrovascular scar by 10 weeks.[11]

In general, many factors have been described to play important roles in the healing pathway, including insulinlike growth factor-1 (IGF-1), vascular endothelial growth factor (VEGF), transforming growth factor beta (TGF-β), platelet-derived growth factor (PDGF) and basic fibroblast growth factor (bFGF).[11] Multiple basic science studies focus on growth factors' effects more specifically on meniscal cells and the processes involved in healing a meniscal tear. Interlukin-1 and epidermal growth factor have been shown to stimulate meniscal cell migration, whereas bone morphogenic proteien-2 and IGF-1 have been shown to stimulate fibrochondrocyte migration from the middle to avascular zone.[12] Webber and coworkers[13] have suggested in their literature that fibroblastic growth factor and human platelet lysate have been found to stimulate the proliferation of meniscal cells. Thus, meniscal repair is based on available vascular supply to supply healing factors. This is the basis for biological enhancement of meniscal repair in avascular areas of the meniscus.

INDICATIONS FOR MENISCAL REPAIR

When a patient presents with knee pain, one should begin with a focused history and physical examination. Specialty tests, such as the McMurray test and Apley grind test, can suggest meniscal pathology, but the most specific physical examination sign suggesting meniscal pathology, as shown by Weinstabl and colleagues al[14], is joint line tenderness in an acutely injured knee. Typical symptoms include pain with deep flexion or twisting, or mechanical symptoms such as an inability to fully extend the knee or the knee locking in certain positions. Imaging studies should begin with radiographs, which include weight-bearing flexion views to identify concomitant osteoarthritis. The most currently effective further imaging study should be a magnetic resonant image. Meniscal tears are treated when they are painful to patients, have failed conservative management, and interfere with daily activities.[14,15]

Indications for repair of meniscal tears are based on several factors, including tear type, location, how acute the tear is, activity level of the patient, patient age, and knee stability. With regard to tear type, the best indication is for unstable tears that are complete and nondegenerative and vertical longitudinal tears greater than 10 to 12 mm in length. Location of meniscal tears is also critical in determining the ability of the tear to heal based on the vascular supply of the meniscus as described above. Tears in the peripheral third are most appropriate for repair because of the excellent blood supply. Repairs of the middle third, the red-white zone, can be attempted as long as they extend into the peripheral third, and central third meniscal tears are generally felt to have poor healing rates as discussed above. Patient-specific factors also play a role in determining if a meniscal tear is appropriate for repair. Active younger patients, in their second, third, or fourth decade of life, are felt to be excellent candidates. Patients also must be willing to undergo postoperative rehabilitation programs as well as adhere to postoperative weight-bearing and activity restrictions. General contra-indications include patients older than 60 years, sedentary lifestyle, unwillingness to participate in postoperative rehabilitation programs or restrictions, or those medically unfit to undergo an operation. Furthermore, degenerative, chronic tears that are stable, less than 10 mm, or in the central third are also contraindicated for repair.[16]

RESULTS

When evaluating meniscal repair results cited in the literature, it is important to consider 3 factors: criteria used to define a successful result, associated injuries, and finally duration of follow-up. Second-look arthroscopy, clinical examinations specific to meniscal symptoms, double-contrast arthrography, and, most recently, magnetic resonance imaging are commonly used to evaluate meniscal repair success. It is important to determine the presence of associated injuries, specifically, anterior cruciate ligament (ACL) rupture, because meniscal repairs associated with ACL tears are frequently more successful based on both the acuteness of injury as well as the presence of a hemarthrosis and associated healing environment the ACL tear creates. Finally, duration of follow-up should be at least 2 years, because shorter follow-up may overestimate success of repair.[17]

In general, meniscal repair rates are more successful for lateral versus medial meniscal tears, when tears are associated with ACL reconstruction, when the rim width is less than 3 mm (peripheral tears), and when tears are results of acute injuries, such as those less than 2 to 8 weeks.[17]

Although the general rule is that meniscal tears of the central third should not be repaired, there are several studies of this that show promise.[2,18,19] In one study by Rubman and colleagues,[20] 198 meniscal tears that initially extended into the avascular zone (rim >4 mm) were repaired and reviewed at least 2 years postoper-atively. Seventy-one percent of the meniscal tears occurred in patients with associ-ated ACL tears. Eighty percent were felt to be asymptomatic for tibiofemoral pain. A total of 91 patients overall were evaluated with follow-up arthroscopy, which showed that 25% were completely healed, 38% partially healed, and 36% did not heal. The authors concluded that meniscal tears into the avascular zone should be repaired because despite the 20% risk of recurrent tibiofemoral symptoms, and 36% overall failure rate on second-look arthroscopy, the benefits of a potentially functional meniscus far outweighed the risk of future degenerative joint arthritis.[20]

Biological Enhancement

Because most studies have found that peripheral meniscal tears heal more predict-ably than central avascular meniscal tears, most effort has been focused on enhancing the potential of healing central meniscal tears. First, mechanical tech-niques, such as rasping[21] and synovial abrasion,[19] were used with some degree of success in an effort to stimulate bleeding and a vascular pannus, which can migrate to the tear and aide in healing by providing inflammatory cells. Recently, biological enhancements, such as fibrin clot, PRP, and growth factors, have been studied, and their application in meniscal repair is discussed below.

Fibrin Clot

Beginning in the 1980s, the literature suggested the use of fibrin clot as an option to adjunct natural healing of meniscal repair. The idea is that by placing a fibrin clot in a stable lesion within the avascular zone of the meniscus, the fibrin clot will aid in healing in 2 ways. First, the fibrin clot will provide a chemotactic and mitogenic stimulus to the reparative process. Furthermore, the fibrin clot itself will serve as scaffolding over which fibrous tissue may from. In a landmark study by Arnoczky and coworkers,[18] avascular tears in the menisci of 6 dogs were surgically created and repaired with the use of a fibrin clot. At 1-, 3-, and 6-month intervals, the menisci were grossly and histologically monitored to check healing status. By 6 months, all of the menisci repaired with fibrin clot were healed grossly and histologically with tissue that resembled mature fibrocartilage, although it did not look like the adjacent uninjured meniscal tissue. Furthermore, the control samples of avascular meniscal tears treated without fibrin clots showed no growth, and in 3 of the 6 samples, only a small film of tissue filled less than 2% of the defect. The key to this technique is not in bringing a direct vascular supply to a previously avascular area, but instead to bring the factors found within a hematoma, which normally forms when there is an injury but cannot form in an avascular meniscal tear. By applying the fibrin clot and the healing factors contained within it, the avascular meniscal repairs have a more natural attempt to heal. In that way the indications for meniscal repair can be broadened, and a larger group of people can benefit from retaining meniscal tissue rather than depending on a menisectomy.[18]

In a study by Henning and colleagues,[19] 153 meniscal tears were repaired with 1 to 2 mL of exogenous fibrin clot. Eight percent of tears were treated in isolation, whereas 92% had association with ACL tear repair. Isolated tears without exogenous clot had a failure rate of 41% compared with 8% when treated with fibrin clot, showing some promise for this treatment option.[19]

Platelet-rich Plasma

PRP is a sample of autologous blood that has been prepared until it has concentrations of platelets that are above baseline values. Higher levels of platelets are desired because studies suggest that growth factors released by platelets recruit reparative cells and may augment soft-tissue repair. PDGF, VEGF, transforming growth factor B1 TGF-β, FGF, and epidermal growth factor have all been found in platelets while hepatocyte growth factor and IGF-1 are found in plasma. These growth factors are important in soft tissue healing, as they induce angiogenesis, stimulate cell replication and differentiation, potentiate other growth factors, and help regulate fibrosis and myocyte regeneration.[22] These growth factors are found in varying concentrations depending on which of the many preparation systems on the market is used.

Preparation of PRP begins as a centrifuge or filter is used to separate the sample of anticoagulated blood into red blood cells, leukocytes, and platelets. The plasma is further concentrated in platelet-rich and platelet-poor portions. Often, the isolated PRP is mixed with an activating agent, such as calcium chloride or thrombin, which creates a putty or gel-like clot, which can then be sutured at the surgical site. These activating agents are used to initiate platelet activation, allowing growth factor release and clot formation at the area of PRP application.[23] As seen in **Fig. 1**, the process of PRP application in meniscal repair includes preparation of the meniscal tear, injection of the PRP gel or putty into the crux of the tear, and repair of meniscus by preferred technique. (See video online for full demonstration of meniscal repair with PRP.)

There are various preparation kits used to create PRP, and each kit results in different proportions of growth factors, activating agent, leukocyte concentration,

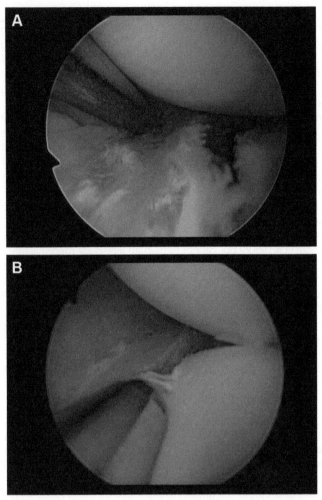

Fig. 1. PRP application to meniscal tear. (*A*) A longitudinal full-thickness meniscal tear is visualized through the arthroscope. (*B*) The meniscal tear has been repaired with edges debrided to a smooth area for repair. The PRP is being injected arthroscopically. The meniscus is then repaired by surgeon preference with PRP within the tear edges.

autologous blood volume, PRP volume, and final platelet amount. Initially, PRP was shown to be clinically effective when the platelet concentration was 4 times that of normal but in further studies has been shown to be effective in lower concentrations. Because of the qualitative and quantitative differences based on preparation kit used to create each lot of PRP, results found in the literature cannot be generalized to all preparation systems.[23]

Before discussing the research that supports PRP use in meniscal tears, it is important to review PRP use in tendon and ligament pathologies—the initial building blocks of why PRP could help in meniscal repair. Basic science studies have found that tendons treated in vivo with PRP showed increased expression of vital reparative growth hormones including VEGF, TGF-β, PDGF compared with those treated with platelet-poor plasma.[24,25] Animal studies have also suggested benefits to PRP use in tendon repair. Murine models with patellar tendon repair enhanced by PRP have shown increased forces to failure, larger tendon callus, and increased tenocyte proliferation.[26,27] Pig ACL reconstruction models enhanced with PRP have shown higher loads to failure, and rabbit patellar tendon repair models have suggested PRP use shows gains in the earlier stages of healing, which appear to level off approximately 4 weeks into the healing process.[28-30] Clinical studies have mainly focused on chronic tendinopathy, such as for lateral epicondylitis and noninsertional Achilles tendonopathy, that has not responded to conservative management. These studies have shown promising results compared with those of placebo (Geaney LE, Arciero RA, DeBerardino TM, et al. The effects of PRP on tendon and ligament: basic science and clinical application. CORR, submitted for publication).[31-33] In the largest randomized, control trial for the use of PRP to treat noninsertional Achilles tendinopathy, no difference was found between the use of PRP and placebo and stretching alone. It has been suggested that these results could be in part because an indication of failure of conservative treatment was not used in the DeVos study.[34]

Thus, basic science and animal studies as well as smaller clinical trials show promising results for PRP in tendon healing, whereas the largest randomized, controlled trial is not as supportive of the use of PRP in tendon healing. The important factors contained in PRP, which show results suggestive of benefit in tendon healing, could also help in the healing process of meniscal repairs in the avascular zone.

Basic science research has suggested that PRP significantly enhances meniscal repair. For example, Ishida and coworkers,[35] in a study performed in Japan, suggested that PRP enhances meniscal tissue regeneration both in vitro and in vivo. They studied mRNA expression of extracellular matrix proteins produced by meniscal cells cultured with PRP compared with meniscal cells without PRP. Significantly higher amounts of mRNA were expressed when cultured with PRP. Even more impressively, in vivo, they showed that full-thickness meniscal tears created in the avascular region of rabbits and treated with PRP delivered by gelatin hydrogel (GH) histologically showed better meniscal repair than those treated with GH and platelet-poor plasma, or GH alone.[35]

There are no large, randomized controlled trials investigating the use of PRP for meniscal repair in human avascular meniscal tears. These studies should be done in future research to contribute to our understanding of the use of PRP in the enhancement of meniscal repair and the expansion of indications for repair.

Tissue Engineering

Cell-based therapy involves growing autologous articular chondrocytes, seeding them to a scaffold, and incorporating this in the repair of meniscal tears. In a study based on a porcine model, this technique resulted in the gross and histologic healing of all specimens. This was in comparison with no repairs seen in the control group, which included 1 meniscal tear repaired with a scaffold alone, 1 with a repair alone, and 1 with no repair at all. Similarly, another porcine-based study showed 100% healing rate with the use of autologous and allogenic chondrocytes seeded on a bioabsorbale mesh and used to treat avascular meniscal tears. This was in comparison with no healing in the control group.[16,36,37] Another idea that has been tested in animal studies is the genetic modification of meniscal and mesenchymal stem cells. These cells were modified to produce TGF-β1, seeded to a scaffold then incorporated in the repair of an avascular meniscal tear in the bovine model. The results showed increased levels of proteogylcan and collagen production as well as histologic evidence of healing.[16,38,39] As these technologies develop, future studies will guide our use of these treatment options in the future.

Growth Factors

The theory of delivering much-needed growth factors to avascular areas of the meniscus is dependent on a good carrier to deliver the growth factors. Because of the short half-life associated with growth factors, it appears that injecting a one-time dose of growth factors would likely be inefficient. Ideally, the scaffold would be a porous, biodegradable material, which could slowly elute growth factors at an effective concentration but would degrade over time as to not interfere with the regenerative process.[40,41] Basic science studies have shown promise for the use of growth factors to stimulate meniscal cells to aid repair of avascular zone meniscal tears. Tumia and colleagues[42] extracted sheep meniscal fibrochondrocytes from the peripheral, middle, and central third of the meniscus, then cultured the cells in fetal calf serum with or without basic FGF and monitored the response of DNA and protein synthesis. The study showed that even cells from the avascular zone responded to bFGF by showing the potential to replicate and produce extracellular matrix.[42]

SUMMARY

The biologic enhancement of meniscal repairs is focused on the delivery of factors that help to create a healing environment despite the lack of natural delivery of these factors in the avascular zone of the meniscus. The use of fibrin clot, PRP, tissue engineering, and local delivery of growth factors are all potential biologic enhancements used in the repair of meniscal tears in the avascular zone of the meniscus. By expanding successful meniscal repair into the avascular zone of the meniscus, many more patients could benefit from this procedure. Larger, randomized studies with human subjects need to be performed to show the potential benefit of these treatment options. Follow-up should be for at least 2 years and can help answer the question whether meniscal repair truly results in the theoretical advantage of avoiding meniscectomy and the associated increased degenerative arthritis that may result.

REFERENCES

1. Annandale T. An operation for displaced semilunar cartilage. Br Med J 1885;1:779.
2. DeHaven K, Arnoczky SP. Meniscal repair. J Bone Joint Surg 1994;43:140–56.
3. Fairbank TJ. Knee joint changes after meniscectomy. J Bone Joint Surg 1948;30B: 664–70.
4. Ahmed AM, Mow VC, Arnoczky S. The load-bearing role of the knee menisci. In: Knee meniscus: basic and clinical foundations. New York: Raven Press; 1992. P. 59–73.
5. Ahmed A, Berke D. In vitro measurement of static pressure distribution in synovial joints—Part I: tibial surface of the knee. J Biomech Eng 1983;105:216–25.
6. Voloshin AS, Wosk J. Shock absorption of meniscectomized and painful knees: a comparative in vivo study. J Biomed Eng 1983;5:157–61.
7. O'Connor BL, McConnaughey JS. The structure and innervation of cat knee menisci, and their relation to a "sensory hypothesis" of meniscal function. Am J Anat 1978; 153:431–42.
8. Wilson A, Legg P, McNeur J. Studies of the innervation of the medial meniscus in the human knee joint. Anat Rec 1969;165:485–91.
9. Bullough P. Munuera L, Murphy J, et al. The strength of the menisci of the knee as it relates to their fine structure. J Bone Joint Surg 1970;52-B(3):564–7.
10. King D. The healing of semilunar cartilages. J Bone Joint Surg 1936;18:1069–76.

11. Arnoczky SP, Warren RF. The microvasculature of the meniscus and its response to injury. An experimental study in the dog. Am J Sports Med 1983;11:131–41.

12. Bhargava MM, Attia ET, Murrell GAC, et al. The effects of cytokines on the proliferation and migration of bovine meniscal cells. Am J Sports Med 1999;27:636–43.

13. Webber RJ, Harris MG, Hough AJ. Cell culture of rabbit meniscal fibrochondrocytes: proliferative and synthetic response to growth factors and ascorbate. J Orthop Res 1985;3:36–42.

14. Weinstabl R, Muellner T, Vecsei V, et al. Economic considerations for the diagnosis and therapy of meniscal lesions: can magnetic resonance imaging help reduce the expense? World J Surg 1997;21:363–8.

15. Greis P, Bardana D, Holmstrom MC. Meniscal injury: I. Basic science and evaluation. J Am Acad Orthop Surg 2002;10:168–76.

16. Noyes F. Barber-Westin S. Repair of complex and avascular meniscal tears and meniscal transplantation. J Bone Joint Surg Am 2010;92:1012–9.

17. Greis P, Holmstrom M, Bardana D, et al. Meniscal injury: II. Management. J Am Acad Orthop Surg 2002;10:177–187.

18. Arnoczky SP, Warren RF, Spivak JM. Meniscal repair using exogenous fibrin clot. An experimental study in dogs. J Bone Joint Surg Am 1988;70:1209–17.

19. Henning CE, Lynch MA, Clark JR. Vascularity for healing meniscus repairs. Arthroscopy 1987;3:13–18.

20. Rubman MH, Noyes FR, Barber-Westin SD. Arthroscopic repair of meniscal tears that extend into the avascular zone: a review of 198 single and complex tears. Am J Sports Med 1998;26:87–95.

21. Okuda K, Ochi M, Shu N, et al. Meniscal rasping for repair of meniscal tear in the avascular zone. Arthroscopy 1999;15:281–6.

22. Eppley BL, Woodell JE, Higgins J. Platelet quantification and growth factor analysis from platelet-rich plasma: implications for wound healing. Plast Reconstr Surg 2004; 114:1502–8.

23. Hall M, Band P, Meislin R, et al. Platelet-rich Plasma: current concepts and application in sports medicine. J Am Acad Orthop Surg 2009;17:602–8.

24. Anitua E, Andia I, Sanchez M, et al. Autologous preparation rich in growth factors promote proliferation and induce VEGF and HGF production by human tendon cells in culture. J Orthop Res 2005;23:281–6.

25. McCarrel T, Fortier L. Temporal growth factor release from platelet-rich plasma, trehalose lyophilized platelets, and bone marrow aspirate and their effect on tendon and ligament gene expression. J Orthop Res 2009;27:1033–42.

26. Aspenberg P, Virchenko O. Platelet concentrate injection improves Achilles tendon repair in rats. Acta Orthop Scand 2004;75:93–9.

27. Kajikawa Y, Morihara T, Sakamoto H, et al. Platelet-rich plasma enhances the initial mobilization of circulation-derived cells for tendon healing. J Cell Physiol 2008;215: 837–45.

28. Flemming BC, Spindler KP, Palmar MP, et al. Collagen-platelet composites improve the biomechanical properties of healing anterior cruciate ligament grafts in a porcine model. Am J Sports Med 2009;37(8):1554–63.

29. Lyras D, Kazakos K, Verettas D, et al. Immunohistochemical study of angiogenesis after local administration of platelet-rich plasma in a patellar tendon defect. Int Orthop 2010;34(1):143–8.

30. Lyras D, Kazakos K, Verettas D, et al. The effect of platelet-rich plasma gel in the early phase of patellar tendon healing. Arch Orthop Trauma Surg 2009;129(11):1577–82.

31. Mirsha A, Pavelko T. Treatment of chronic elbow tendinosis with buffered platelet-rich plasma. Am J Sports Med 2006;34(11):1774–8.

32. Peerbooms J, Sluimer J, Bruinj D, et al. Positive effect of an autologous platelet concentrate in lateral epicondylitis in a double-blind randomized controlled trial: platelet-rich plasma versus corticosteroid injection with a 1-year follow-up. Am J Sports Med 2010;38(2):255–62.

33. Gaweda K, Tarczynska M, Krzyanowki W. Treatment of Achilles tendinopathy with platelet-rich plasma. Int J Sports Med 2010;31(8):577–83.

34. De Vos RJ, Weir A, Van Schie HTM, et al. Platelet-rich plasma injection for chronic Achilles tendinopathy: a randomized controlled trial. JAMA 2010;303(2):144–9.

35. Ishida K, Kuroda R, Miwa M, et al. The regenerative effects of platelet-rich plasma on meniscal cells in vitro and in vivo application with biodegradable gelatin hydrogel. Tiss Eng 2007;13(5):1103–12.

36. Peretti GM, Gill TJ, Xu JW, et al. Cell-based therapy for meniscal repair: a large animal study. Am J Sports Med 2004;32:146–58.

37. Weinand C, Peretti GM, Adams SB Jr, et al. An allogenic cell-based implant for meniscal lesions. Am J Sports Med 2006;34:1779–89.

38. Izuta Y, Ochi M, Adachi N, et al. Meniscal repair using bone marrow-derived mesenchymal stem cells: experimental study using green fluorescent protein transgenic rats. Knee 2005;12:217–23.

39. Steinert AF, Palmer GD, Capito R, et al. Genetically enhanced engineering of meniscus tissue using ex vivo delivery of transofmring growth factor-β1 complementary deoxyribonucleic acid. Tiss Eng 2007;13:227–37.

40. Forriol F. Growth factors in cartilage and meniscus repair. Injury 2009;40:12–16.

41. Hidaka C, Ibarra C, Hannafin JA, et al: Formation of vascularized meniscal tissue by combining gene therapy with engineering. Tiss Eng 2002;8:93–105.

42. Tumia NS, Johnstone AJ. Promoting the proliferative and synthetic acitivty of knee meniscal fibrochondrocytes using basic fibroblast growth factor in vitro. Am J Sports Med 2004;32:915–20.

Meniscus Root Avulsion

John M. Marzo, MD

KEYWORDS

• Meniscus • Root • Tear • Avulsion • Repair

Root tears of the menisci were underappreciated as a clinical entity until a case report by Pagnani and coworkers,[1] who described a medial meniscal root tear in a young athlete. This case and others in subsequent reports were managed by partial meniscectomy because they were felt to be irreparable or degenerative in origin or because techniques for repair had not yet been described.[2–5] At the same time, as repair techniques began to appear in the literature, basic science, radiologic, and biomechanical studies supported the rational for doing so.[6–12] There are now several case series that report the clinical, radiologic, and second-look arthroscopic results of meniscal root repair.[11,13–16] The majority of the available literature pertains to medial meniscal root tears, but there are some reports regarding lateral meniscal root tears.[17–22] This article, like other reviews, summarizes what is currently known about this condition with emphasis on the medial meniscal root, but most of the concepts seem applicable to the lateral meniscus as well.[23,24] Current consensus is that meniscal root tears should be clinically recognized, and strong consideration should be given to surgical repair in selected cases by utilizing 1 of several reported techniques designed to anatomically restore the root, maximize meniscal function, and preserve the heath of the knee joint.

EPIDEMIOLOGY

There is a bimodal distribution of patients with meniscal root tears, a smaller peak in young patients who sustain trauma, and a larger peak in middle-age patients who more likely suffer from attritional degenerative radial tearing.[13,15,25] In the second and larger peak, the average age is 52 to 55 years, and there is a higher incidence in Far Eastern people as well as an association with obesity.[13,25,26] At the time of arthroscopy for suspected medial meniscal problems, studies have reported radial tear at or adjacent to the meniscal root or root avulsion in between 1% and 28% of cases.[5,25,27–29] In a study by Brody and colleagues,[19] of 264 patients who sustained an ACL tear, 9.8% had a lateral meniscal root tear and 3% had a medial meniscal root tear. In a similar study of 365 patients with ACL, posterior cruciate ligament (PCL), or

The author has nothing to disclose.

Department of Orthopaedic Surgery, State University of New York, University at Buffalo, 160 Farber Hall, Main Street, Buffalo, New York 14214, USA

E-mail address: jmmarzo@buffalo.edu

Clin Sports Med 31 (2012) 101–111

doi:10.1016/j.csm.2011.08.013

0278-5919/12/$ – see front matter © 2012 Elsevier Inc. All rights reserved.

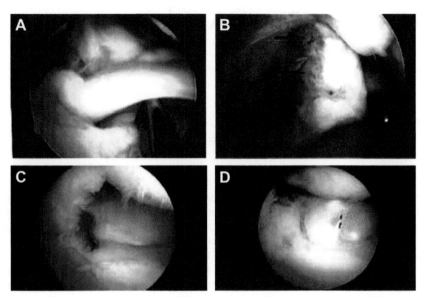

Fig. 1. (*A*) Arthroscopic appearance of a normal medial meniscal root attachment. (*B*) arthroscopic appearance of a boney avulsion of the meniscal root. (*From* Marzo JM. Medial meniscus posterior horn avulsion. J Am Acad Orthop Surg 2009;17(5):276–83; with permission.) (*C*) Arthroscopic appearance of a medial meniscal root avulsion. (*D*) Arthroscopic appearance of a repaired medial meniscal root.

combined ligament injured knees, Kim and coworkers[15] found the same incidence of 3% medial meniscal root tear.

CLINICAL PRESENTATION AND DIAGNOSIS

The typical presentation of a patient with a meniscal root tear is much like any patient with a meniscal tear, with 2 notable exceptions: more severe pain than usual, and more abrupt onset.[5] In the series of patients reported by Beasley and colleagues,[4] 74% of patients reported a specific mechanism of injury, whereas 26% reported an insidious onset of symptoms. Habata and coworkers[5] reported that 85% of patients could recall a discreet event that preceded a chief complaint of pain. Some of our patients have described a sense of walking as if "bone on bone" when trying to describe how they feel after a meniscal root avulsion. Physical examination findings usually include a knee effusion, medial joint line tenderness, diminished knee flexion, and a positive pain response with McMurray test.[5,13,25,28] Plain radiographs are usually normal in younger patients but one should be aware of the possibility of a bony avulsion of the meniscal root, which may be seen as a "meniscal ossicle" (**Fig. 1A, B**).[3,6,8] Radiographs may only show evidence of mild to moderate degenerative changes in the older patient group. Magnetic resonance imaging (MRI) is the imaging modality of choice, and the features of a medial meniscal avulsion are quite characteristic.[30] The normal meniscal root is visible in all planes as a low signal band of tissue extending from the posterior horn of the meniscus to its attachment on the tibia, just in front of the posterior cruciate ligament. The described features of a root avulsion include the meniscal ghost sign (absence of the meniscus on the sagittal view), the presence of radial tear on coronal and occasionally on axial slices, and

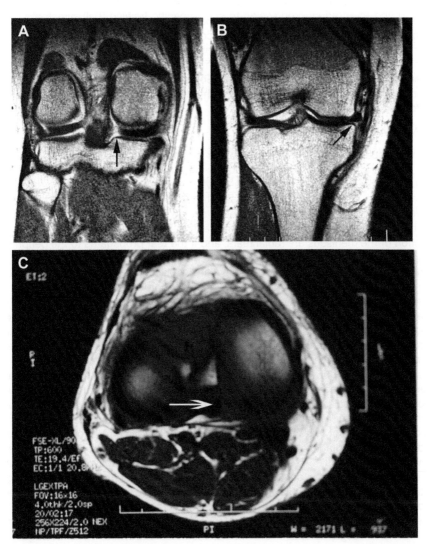

Fig. 2. (A) Coronal MR image at the level of the medial meniscal root shows a gap (*arrow*) where the meniscus has avulsed and separated from the tibia. (B) MR image of the same patient at the midcoronal tibial level shows medial meniscal extrusion of greater than 3 mm (*arrow*), measured as the difference between one vertical line drawn at the medial edge of the tibial plateau at the transition from vertical to horizontal and a second vertical line drawn from the medial margin of the medial meniscus. (C) MR axial image that illustrates the medial meniscus avulsed with a gap (*arrow*) between the normal root attachment and the meniscus.

perhaps most important, evidence of meniscus extrusion >3 mm on midcoronal cuts (**Fig. 2**).[2,29,31] Meniscal extrusion is a very important (albeit not specific) sign of the possibility of a meniscal root tear and has been associated with medial joint space narrowing, sclerosis, and the signs of degenerative arthritis on MRI scan.[2,32–35] Brody and coworkers[19] noted that when lateral meniscus extrusion was seen on MRI, 88% were associated with meniscal root avulsion. At the time of diagnostic arthroscopy, the surgeon must include an inspection and probing of the medial meniscus root, which is best visualized by placing the scope into and through the intercondylar notch, between the posterior aspect of the medial wall of the femur and the posterior cruciate ligament (**Fig. 1**C). For this maneuver, the knee is best positioned in extension while valgus stress is exerted. Some surgeons may prefer to use a 70° arthroscope at this time, similar to when the tibial side of a PCL reconstruction is performed.

BIOMECHANICS

It is well accepted that the meniscus serves to function as a main shock absorber of the knee and to more evenly distribute load through the knee joint.[36,37] The circumferential fibers of the meniscus provide resistance to hoop stress, avoiding radial expansion or extrusion by being strongly anchored at the anterior and posterior roots. Deficiency of the meniscus has been shown to increase loads across the joint in studies of both partial and total meniscectomy.[38] Particularly deleterious to the function of the meniscus are radial tears, and if the tear propagates to the peripheral rim, the result is a mechanical effect similar to that of total meniscectomy.[32,33,35,39–41] Further models show that complete radial tears involving the posterior one-third of the meniscus render the meniscus unable to absorb hoop stress, and meniscus transplants that are not firmly attached at the root illustrate a loading profile similar to that of a complete meniscectomy in cadaveric studies.[42,43] In a laboratory biomechanical study specific to the topic of this review, the consequence of an avulsion of the posterior root of the medial meniscus is to increase joint load, decrease joint contact area, and result in an increased peak pressure in the medial compartment of 25%.[10] A similar study in our laboratory showed an increase in medial tibiofemoral peak pressure of 24%, and a decrease in contact area of 20%.[9] Importantly, both studies showed that repair of the experimental root avulsion through a transosseous technique resulted in loading profiles returning to normal. A single animal study of medial meniscal root tears confirmed increased medial tibiofemoral contact pressure and decreased contact area from flexion of 30° to 90°, but contact pressure was still elevated at 0° to 30°.[44] This might raise concern about the repair during the stance phase of gait and give some caution regarding postoperative motion or weight bearing.[44] Meniscal root avulsions are, in effect, complete radial tears and have been shown to cause meniscus extrusion in radiographic and laboratory studies.[2,32,45–47] A recent biomechanical laboratory study found that the immediate effect of a medial root avulsion is gap creation and medial meniscal extrusion.[45] The average gap measured 4.7 mm in the unloaded knee and increased to 7.0 mm when the knee was under a physiologic load of 1800 N. At the midcoronal position, the meniscus extruded an average of 3.28 mm under load, and repair restored ability of the meniscus to resist extrusion under the same load (average of only 1.46 mm; $P<.001$). To date, there are no studies of the behavior of experimental meniscal root avulsions under cyclic loading conditions.

There has been a strong association of meniscus extrusion with the presence of osteoarthritis; enough to support the contention that there is a direct relationship between meniscus root avulsion, meniscus extrusion, and degenerative arthritis.[35,39,48–50] Some studies report that femorotibial degenerative arthritis is not present in a subset of cases of medial meniscal extrusion, suggesting that meniscal root tear may precede and predispose to the development of arthritis.[31,35,39] It is still uncertain, however, whether meniscal extrusion is the cause of arthritis or a byproduct of arthritis. In another possible subset of patients, Robertson and coworkers[51] recently published a series of 30 patients in whom spontaneous osteonecrosis of the medial femoral condyle developed and noted an associated medial meniscal root tear by MRI in 80% of this group. While not claiming a cause and effect relationship, this interesting phenomenon deserves further study.

TREATMENT OPTIONS AND RESULTS

Nonoperative care of patients with this condition can be considered when symptoms are minimal or future activity demands are limited. Supportive measures include activity avoidance or modification, weight loss when appropriate, modalities, and medical/pharmaceutical or neutriceutical management. Soft shock-absorbing footwear, rear-posted wedge shoe orthotics, and unloader braces all have some theoretical mechanical advantage and can be tried, especially in cases in which there is some preexisting malalignment. Nonoperative care of patients with posterior meniscal root avulsions can be successful, and clinical studies show improvement up to 12 months that then decline but remain improved over initial scores for up to 36 months later.[26]

Surgical options include arthroscopic partial meniscectomy or arthroscopic-assisted meniscal root repair. Patients with root tears that are considered irreparable in an otherwise normal knee (thought to be an unusual combination) may be candidates for meniscal transplantation. Also to be considered while planning a meniscal root repair is correction of instability or malalignment, another topic beyond the scope of this review. Partial meniscectomy is indicated when the meniscus is of poor quality in holding repair sutures, when the meniscus will not reduce to the root location on the tibia, or if the knee joint already has significant chondral disease. These criteria may preclude many patients from repair, as there is a known association of an attritional root tear, extrusion, and degenerative disease in as many as 80% of this group when MRIs are analyzed.[2,33,35] Another reason to accept partial meniscectomy as an option is when the patient cannot, or is unwilling to, participate in the required postoperative protective weight bearing and prolonged rehabilitation. Several clinical studies have reported that subjective symptoms improve significantly after arthroscopic partial meniscectomy.[5,15,25,28] This especially seems to be the case when the patient has mechanical symptoms relative to the tear as the chief preoperative clinical complaint. Han and colleagues,[14] on the other hand, state that although partial meniscectomy significantly improved postoperative Lysholm clinical scores, only 56% had improvement in pain, 67% were satisfied with the outcome, and 35% showed radiographic progression of osteoarthritis at a mean of 77 months of follow-up. They note a significant negative correlation between chondral wear at arthroscopy and postoperative modified Lysholm knee score. In a random sampling of 67 patients who underwent arthroscopic partial medial meniscectomy for radial tears at the meniscal root, Ozkoc and coworkers[25] found a modest improvement in Lysholm score (53 to 67) but increased postoperative Kellgren-Lawrence scores showing a significant worsening of radiographic grade of arthritis. Neither nonoperative treatment nor arthroscopic partial meniscectomy would seem have a positive effect on what is thought to be the mechanical cascade of meniscal root tear, meniscus extrusion, and progressive osteoarthritis.

Many surgical techniques to repair the meniscal root have been described in the literature, all designed to reduce and fix the meniscal root to a prepared bony bed at the location of the root attachment (see **Fig. 1**).[3,7,8,11,12,22,52–54] The clearest indication for meniscal root repair is in a young patient at the time of ligament surgery or in any patient with an isolated root tear and a well-preserved knee joint. In all other cases, the surgeon must make a critical assessment of the amount of chondral disease that is present and decide if root restoration alone or in combination with joint restoration would be theoretically beneficial and be tolerated by the patient. The average age of the patients in the second peak in occurrence in our study was 55 years. Therefore, absolute age does not seem to be the determining factor for repairing the meniscus, rather, it is the condition of the articular surfaces of the knee In a comparison study by Kim and colleagues,16 arthroscopic pull-out repair of a medial meniscal root tear gave significantly better clinical and radiologic results than partial meniscectomy, and sound healing of the meniscus with restoration of hoop tension was observed by MRI and at second-look arthroscopy. Many case reports and small clinical series report favorable results of various repair techniques, and recently there have been reports with larger numbers of patients and longer periods of follow-up.[11,13,15,16,21,55] In separate retrospective reviews, Ahn and coworkers[21] and Anderson and coworkers[56] have confirmed reliable healing of posterior horn lateral meniscal root repairs when performed in combination with ACL reconstruction. The report by Seo and colleagues,[13] while showing improved clinical outcome in 21 patients, calls into question the ability of the meniscus to heal based on gross findings at second-look arthroscopy. Of 11 patients during second-look arthroscopy, they found none with complete healing: 5 had lax healing, 4 had scar tissue healing, and 2 had failed healing. Separate studies by Kim and colleagues[15] and Lee and colleagues[55] also showed improved clinical results and comparatively better rates of healing as shown by MRI or second-look arthroscopy. In the study by Lee and colleagues,[55] preoperative Lysholm score improved from 57 to 93 at follow-up of at least 2 years, and they reported complete healing in all 10 patients who underwent second-look arthros-copy.[55]

TECHNICAL PEARLS FOR MEDIAL MENISCAL ROOT REPAIR AND REHABILITATION

The majority of the reported techniques demand a certain skill driving the arthro-scope, using accessory portals, and navigating around the knee joint to optimize visualization of the root attachment. An excellent description of 1 common technique using transosseous sutures can be found in a recent review by Harner and cowork-ers[57] and is complete with diagrams and intra-articular photos. A technical report by Choi and colleagues[58] describes the use of suture anchors and sutures in a method similar to rotator cuff repair. An accessory posteromedial portal can be very useful for preparing the meniscal root and the tibial root attachment site, passing sutures and anchors, and tying arthroscopic knots for certain of the techniques of repair. It may also be helpful for creating a central transpatellar tendon portal for the arthroscope or for furthering aid in manipulation of the meniscal root and repair sutures. It is advisable to perform a mini-notchplasty to remove the medial aspect of the tibial spine and occasionally the posteromedial aspect of the lateral wall of the medial femur to improve visualization of the surgical site and to increase room for carrying out the repair. Fat and synovium along the inferior portion of the PCL can also be resected to enhance visualization. Our preferred technique is to use a transtibial tunnel patterned after a procedure first described by Shino and colleagues[59] and then by West and colleagues[22] to repair lateral meniscal root tears, which has evolved to the use of suture lasso devices rather than larger suture-passing devices referred to in the original report (**Fig. 3**).[7] The tibial socket technique, however, is particularly useful when repairing a meniscal root at the same time as cruciate ligament reconstruction, as it helps avoid the potential problem of tunnel coalescence.[53] We still prefer the transosseous tunnel technique because the tunnel itself becomes useful as another working portal for suture-passing devices and for placement of

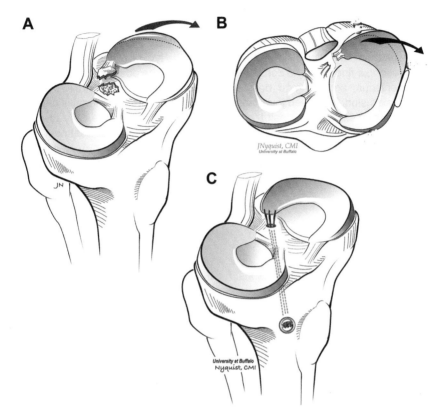

Fig. 3. Schematic drawings depict a medial meniscal ossicle (*A*), a medial meniscal avulsion (*B*), and a medial meniscal root repair by the transtibial tunnel method (*C*). (**Figs. 3***B, C From* Marzo JM. Medial meniscus posterior horn avulsion. J Am Acad Orthop Surg 2009;17(5):276–83; with permission.)

repair sutures.[7] It should be recognized that simple vertical and horizontal sutures are weaker in the meniscus than Kessler, Krackow, Mason-Allen, or other types of suture/soft tissue configurations. Only open techniques allow tying of the more complicated sutures, and this may prove to be a relative weakness of the current arthroscopic fixation techniques.

The strength of the different repair techniques is not known, and there are no studies of the abilities of the repairs under cyclic loading, so it remains prudent to protect the knee from weight bearing and excessive motion during the early postoperative period. A hinged knee brace set to allow 0° to 45° of knee flexion is applied in the operating room. Active straight leg raises, quadriceps sets, hip exercises, and calf pumps are started on the first postoperative day. The patient is non–weight bearing with crutches for the first 4 weeks, then advanced from touch-down weight bearing to full over the next 2 weeks. The brace is unlocked 0° to 90° at 2 weeks and heel slides and active knee flexion begun, advancing gradually to 90° until 4 weeks, and advanced as tolerated thereafter. Use of the brace and crutches can be discontinued after 6 weeks and when the patient has good leg control.

SUMMARY

Meniscal root radial tears and avulsions occur frequently enough that one should be familiar with them as a clinical entity and recognize the typical clinical symptoms, MRI, and arthroscopic findings. The consequence of loss of the posterior horn attachment of the meniscus, according to best evidence, is loss of hoop strain constraint, meniscus extrusion, increased joint pressure, and premature degenerative disease of the knee over time. Surgical repair techniques are available, and the early-to-middle-range clinical results seem superior to those of nonoperative treatment or arthroscopic partial meniscectomy. Further basic and clinical studies are necessary to examine the effect of repair on the mechanics of the knee under cyclic loading and on the long-term clinical outcome.

REFERENCES

1. Pagnani MJ, Cooper DE, Warren RF. Extrusion of the medial meniscus. Arthroscopy 1991;7(3):297–300.
2. Jones AO, Houang MT, Low RS, et al. Medial meniscus posterior root attachment injury and degeneration: MRI findings. Australas Radiol 2006;50(4):306–13.
3. Berg EE. The meniscal ossicle: the consequence of a meniscal avulsion. Arthroscopy 1991;7(2):241–3.
4. Beasley L, Robertson D, Armfeld D. Medial meniscal root tears: demographic, radiographic, and arthroscopic findings. The Pittsburgh Orthopedic Journal 2005;6: 155.
5. Habata T, Uematsu K, Hattori K, et al. Clinical features of the posterior horn tear in the medial meniscus. Arch Orthop Trauma Surg 2004;124(9):642–5.
6. Griffith CJ, LaPrade RF, Fritts HM, et al. Posterior root avulsion fracture of the medial meniscus in an adolescent female patient with surgical reattachment. Am J Sports Med 2008;36(4):789–92.
7. Marzo JM, Kumar BA. Primary repair of medial meniscal avulsions—2 case studies. Am J Sports Med 2007;35(8):1380–3.
8. Raustol OA, Poelstra KA, Chhabra A, et al. The meniscal ossicle revisited: etiology and an arthroscopic technique for treatment. Arthroscopy 2006;22(6):687,681–3.
9. Marzo JM, Gurske-DePerio J. Effects of medial meniscus posterior horn avulsion and repair on tibiofemoral contact area and peak contact pressure with clinical implications. Am J Sports Med 2009;37(1):124–9.
10. Allaire R, Muriuki M, Gilbertson L, et al. Biomechanical consequences of a tear of the posterior root of the medial meniscus. Similar to total meniscectomy. J Bone Joint Surg Am 2008;90(9):1922–31.
11. Jones C, Reddy S, Ma CB. Repair of the posterior root of the medial meniscus. Knee 2010;17(1):77–80.
12. Kim YM, Rhee KJ, Lee JK, et al. Arthroscopic pullout repair of a complete radial tear of the tibial attachment site of the medial meniscus posterior horn. Arthroscopy 2006;22(7):795A-U748.
13. Seo HS, Lee SC, Jung KA. Second-look arthroscopic findings after repairs of posterior root tears of the medial meniscus. Am J Sports Med 2011;39(1):99–107.
14. Han SB, Shetty GM, Lee DH, et al. Unfavorable results of partial meniscectomy for complete posterior medial meniscus root tear with early osteoarthritis: a 5- to 8-year follow-up study. Arthroscopy 2010;26(10):1326–32.
15. Kim YJ, Kim JG, Chang SH, et al. Posterior root tear of the medial meniscus in multiple knee ligament injuries. Knee 2010;17(5):324–8.

16. Kim SB, Ha JK, Lee SW, et al. Medial meniscus root tear refixation: comparison of clinical, radiologic, and arthroscopic findings with medial meniscectomy. Arthroscopy 2011;27(3):346–54.
17. Kenny C. Arthroscopic repair of avulsion of the posterior root and body of the lateral meniscus: a twenty-year follow-up. A case report. J Bone Joint Surg Am 2009;91(12): 2932–6.
18. Petersen W, Zantop T. Avulsion injury to the posterior horn of the lateral meniscus. Technique for arthroscopic refixation. Unfallchirurg 2006;109(11):984–7.
19. Brody JM, Lin HM, Hulstyn MJ, et al. Lateral meniscus root tear and meniscus extrusion with anterior cruciate ligament tear. Radiology 2006;239(3):805–10.
20. Ahn JH, Lee YS, Yoo JC, et al. Results of arthroscopic all-inside repair for lateral meniscus root tear in patients undergoing concomitant anterior cruciate ligament reconstruction. Arthroscopy 2010;26(1):67–75.
21. Ahn JH, Lee YS, Chang JY, et al. Arthroscopic all inside repair of the lateral meniscus root tear. Knee 2009;16(1):77–80.
22. West RV, Kim JG, Armfield D, et al. Lateral meniscal root tears associated with anterior cruciate ligament injury: classification and management (SS-70). Arthroscopy 2004;20(Suppl 1):e32–3.
23. Marzo JM. Medial meniscus posterior horn avulsion. J Am Acad Orthop Surg 2009;17(5):276–83.
24. Koenig JH, Ranawat AS, Umans HR, et al. Meniscal root tears: diagnosis and treatment. Arthroscopy 2009;25(9):1025–32.
25. Ozkoc G, Circi E, Gonc U, et al. Radial tears in the root of the posterior horn of the medial meniscus. Knee Surg Sports Traumatol Arthrosc 2008;16(9):849–54.
26. Lim HC, Bae JH, Wang JH, et al. Non-operative treatment of degenerative posterior root tear of the medial meniscus. Knee Surg Sports Traumatol Arthrosc 2010;18(4): 535–39.
27. Kidron A, Thein R. Radial tears associated with cleavage tears of the medial meniscus in athletes. Arthroscopy 2002;18(3):254–6.
28. Bin SI, Kim JM, Shin SJ. Radial tears of the posterior horn of the medial meniscus. Arthroscopy 2004;20(4):373–8.
29. Harper KW, Helms CA, Lambert HS III, et al. Radial meniscal tears: significance, incidence, and MR appearance. Am J Roentgenol 2005;185(6):1429–34.
30. So YL, Jee WH, Kim JM. Radial tear of the medial meniscal root: reliability and accuracy of MRI for diagnosis. Am J Roentgenol 2008;191(1):81–5.
31. Lee YG, Shim JC, Choi YS, et al. Magnetic resonance imaging findings of surgically proven medial meniscus root tear: tear configuration and associated knee abnormalities. J Comput Assist Tomogr 2008;32(3):452–7.
32. Kenny C. Radial displacement of the medial meniscus and Fairbank's signs. Clin Orthop Relat Res 1997(339):163–73.
33. Costa CR, Morrison WB, Carrino JA. Medial meniscus extrusion on knee MRI: is extent associated with severity of degeneration or type of tear? AJR Am J Roentgenol 2004;183(1):17–23.
34. Boxheimer L, Lutz AM, Treiber K, et al. MR imaging of the knee: position related changes of the menisci in asymptomatic volunteers. Invest Radiol 2004;39(5): 254–63.
35. Lerer DB, Umans HR, Xu MX, et al. The role of meniscal root pathology and radial meniscal tear in medial meniscal extrusion. Skeletal Radiol 2004;33(10):569–74.
36. Wojtys EM, Chan DB. Meniscus structure and function. Instructional course lectures 2005;54:323–30.

37. Renstrom P, Johnson RJ. Anatomy and biochechanics of the menisci. Clin Sports Med 1990;9(3):523–38.
38. McBride ID, Reid JG. Biomechanical considerations of the menisci of the knee. Canadian journal of sport sciences = Journal canadien des sciences du sport 1988; 13(4):175–87.
39. Gale DR, Chaisson CE, Totterman SMS, et al. Meniscal subluxation: association with osteoarthritis and joint space narrowing. Osteoarthritis Cartilage 1999;7(6):526–32.
40. Sugita T, Kawamata T, Ohnuma M, et al. Radial displacement of the medial meniscus in varus osteoarthritis of the knee. Clin Orthop Relat Res 2001(387):171–7.
41. Lee SJ, Aadalen KJ, Malaviya P, et al. Tibiofemoral contact mechanics after serial medial meniscectomies in the human cadaveric knee. Am J Sports Med 2006;34(8): 1334–44.
42. Spencer Jones R, Keene GCR, Learmonth DJA, et al. Direct measurement of hoop strains in the intact and torn human medial meniscus. Clinl Biomech 1996;11(5):295–300.
43. Paletta GA Jr, Manning T, Snell E, et al. The effect of allograft meniscal replacement on intraarticular contact area and pressures in the human knee. A biomechanical study. Am J Sports Med 1997;25(5):692–8.
44. Seo JH, Li G, Shetty GM, et al. Effect of repair of radial tears at the root of the posterior horn of the medial meniscus with the pullout suture technique: a biomechanical study using porcine knees. Arthroscopy 2009;25(11):1281–7.
45. Hein CN, Deperio JG, Ehrensberger MT, et al. Effects of medial meniscal posterior horn avulsion and repair on meniscal displacement. Knee 2011;18(3):189–92.
46. Rennie WJ, Finlay DBL. Meniscal extrusion in young athletes: associated knee joint abnormalities. Am J Roentgenol 2006;186(3):791–4.
47. Choi CJ, Choi YJ, Lee JJ, et al. Magnetic resonance imaging evidence of meniscal extrusion in medial meniscus posterior root tear. Arthroscopy 2010;26(12):1602–6.
48. Kan A, Oshida M, Oshida S, et al. Anatomical significance of a posterior horn of medial meniscus: the relationship between its radial tear and cartilage degradation of joint surface. Sports Med Arthrosc Rehabil Ther Technol 2010;2:1.
49. Pelletier JP, Raynauld JP, Berthiaume MJ, et al. Risk factors associated with the loss of cartilage volume on weight-bearing areas in knee osteoarthritis patients assessed by quantitative magnetic resonance imaging: a longitudinal study. Arthritis Research and Therapy 2007;9(4).
50. Berthiaume MJ, Raynauld JP, Martel-Pelletier J, et al. Meniscal tear and extrusion are strongly associated with progression of symptomatic knee osteoarthritis as assessed by quantitative magnetic resonance imaging. Ann Rheum Dis 2005;64(4):556–63.
51. Robertson DD, Armfield DR, Towers JD, et al. Meniscal root injury and spontaneous osteonecrosis of the knee: an observation. J Bone Joint Surg Br 2009;91(2):190–5.
52. Richmond JC, Sarno RC. Arthroscopic treatment of medial meniscal avulsion fractures. Arthroscopy 1988;4(2):117–20.
53. Nicholas SJ, Golant A, Schachter AK, et al. A new surgical technique for arthroscopic repair of the meniscus root tear. Knee Surg Sports Traumatol Arthrosc 2009;17(12): 1433–6.
54. Engelsohn E, Umans H, DiFelice GS. Marginal fractures of the medial tibial plateau: possible association with medial meniscal root tear. Skeletal Radiol 2007;36(1):73–6.
55. Lee JH, Lim YJ, Kim KB, et al. Arthroscopic pullout suture repair of posterior root tear of the medial meniscus: radiographic and clinical results with a 2-year follow-up. Arthroscopy 2009;25(9):951–8.

56. Anderson L, Watts M, Shapter O, et al. Repair of radial tears and posterior horn detachments of the lateral meniscus: minimum 2-year follow-up. Arthroscopy 2010; 26(12):1625–1632+e1212.
57. Harner CD, Mauro CS, Lesniak BP, et al. Biomechanical consequences of a tear of the posterior root of the medial meniscus. Surgical technique. J Bone Joint Surg Am 2009;91 Suppl 2:257–70.
58. Choi NH, Son KM, Victoroff BN. Arthroscopic all-inside repair for a tear of posterior root of the medial meniscus: a technical note. Knee Surg Sports Traumatol Arthrosc 2008;16(9):891–3.
59. Shino K, Hamada M, Mitsuoka T, et al. Case report: arthroscopic repair for a flap tear of the posterior horn of the lateral meniscus adjacent to its tibial insertion. Arthroscopy 1995;11(4):495–8.

Posterior Horn Tears— All-Inside Suture Repair

Jin Hwan Ahn, MD[a], Jae Chul Yoo, MD[b], Sang Hak Lee, MD[c],*

KEYWORDS

- Meniscus tear • Posterior horn • Repair • All-inside suture

As our understanding of meniscus function has improved, meniscal repair represents the standard for treatment of vertical meniscal tears within the vascularized zone, where healing can be biologically expected.[1,2] However, surgical repair may be technically demanding and time-consuming. Although the conventional repair methods, including arthroscopic inside-out and outside-in suture techniques, are considered the gold standard,[3–6] they have the risk of inadvertent neurovascular injury, require additional skin incisions, and can be technically cumbersome.[7,8] The introduction of all-inside devices has been a turning point in the advance of arthroscopic technique because of simplicity of implant insertion and the reduction in surgery time.[9–12] However, recent studies suggest potential problems with all-inside devices, such as nonanatomic coaptation, loss of fixation, aseptic synovitis, and inadvertent chondral injury.[13–16] In addition, significantly lower resistance to load bearing compared with traditional vertical sutures has been reported, although its clinical importance is not known.[17–19] Most importantly, all-inside devices are relatively contraindicated for tears near the meniscocapsular junction and lateral meniscus (LM) popliteal hiatus because it has weak holding strength.

All-inside meniscal suturing, which Morgan[20] first described, allows placement of vertically oriented sutures, which have the strongest pullout strength.[21] However, Morgan's technique of all-inside suturing has several disadvantages, such as fluid extravasation through the required 8-mm cannula, which causes loss of articular distension; a restricted area available for meniscus suture that consists of approximately 3 mm of the meniscocapsular junction; and more technical difficulty in manipulating the suture hook through a single cannula. As an alternative, we previously reported an arthroscopic modified all-inside suture

The authors have nothing to disclose.

[a] Department of Orthopaedic Surgery, Sungkyunkwan University, School of Medicine, Kangbuk Samsung Hospital, 108, Pyoung-Dong, Jongro-Ku, Seoul, 110-746, Korea
[b] Department of Orthopaedic Surgery, Samsung Medical Center, Sungkyunkwan University, School of Medicine, 50 Ilwon-Dong, Kangnam-Ku, Seoul, 135-710, Korea
[c] Department of Orthopaedic Surgery, Center for Joint Diseases and Rheumatism, Kyung Hee University Hospital at Gangdong, 892 Dongnam-ro, Gangdong-gu, Seoul, 134-727, Korea
* Corresponding author.
E-mail address: sangdory@hanmail.net

technique of Morgan using 2 posteromedial (PM) portals for repair of medial meniscus posterior horn (MMPH) tears.[22,23] However, recently we began performing arthroscopic all-inside suture for posterior horn tear of medial or LM through a single PM or posterolateral (PL) portal.[24] Our suturing technique allows greater freedom in suture hook maneuvering by creating a single posterior portal without using a cannula. This technique allows excellent visualization of the posterior compartment, anatomic coaptation of the torn meniscus, and strong knot tying, while avoiding inadvertent injury to the remnant meniscus and articular cartilage. The indication for this repair technique is both longitudinal tears being within 5 mm of peripheral rim and greater than 1 cm in size at posterior horn of both menisci. In addition, radial tears, involving the red-white or red-red zone in the midbody or root of the LM, were considered indications for all-inside meniscal suturing.

SURGICAL TECHNIQUE
Longitudinal Tear of Medial Meniscus Posterior Horn

Up to two-thirds of patients with anterior cruciate ligament (ACL) rupture have combined MMPH tears.[25–29] Repairing this torn meniscus anatomically allows the reconstructed ACL knee to be more stable than those repaired with a meniscectomy.[30] However, many surgeons overlook this combined tear because of its concealing location and benign appearance from the anterior portals. Furthermore, MMPH peripheral rim tears may heal slowly despite the rich vascular supply to the red-red zone, because a torn meniscus has some vertical movement superiorly against the meniscocapsular junction.[23,31,32] A recent clinical study found that the rate of poor results for repair of MM tears remained high when conservative treatment

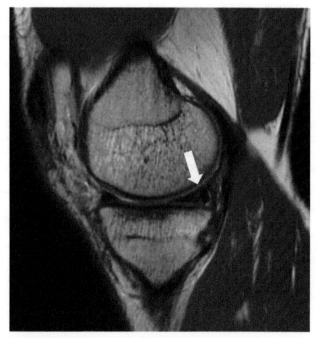

Fig. 1. The sagittal MRI finding shows longitudinal tear of posterior horn of medial meniscus (*arrow*).

was used, even though the conservative approach was more effective for LM.[32,33] Previous studies have found that magnetic resonance imaging (MRI) has a sensitivity of only 69% to 89% for detecting meniscal tears in patients with acute or chronic ACL tears.[34–36] With the advent of higher-resolution MRI scans, most of peripheral MMPH tears associated with an ACL injury can be detected on the sagittal plane of the MRI (**Fig. 1**).

Diagnostic arthroscopy

Allowing adequate room for placement of the posterior portals and space for maneuvering the intra-articular instruments is imperative when positioning the patient. The opposite healthy limb is elevated in a lithotomy position. The injured knee should be flexed 90° by hanging down at the edge of operating table, which allows distention of the posterior compartments. Also, this position permits manipulation of intra-articular instruments with relative ease and simultaneously protects the saphenous nerve by displacing it well posterior from the joint line. The standard anterolateral (AL) and anteromedial (AM) portals are used for comprehensive examination with a 30° arthroscope and a probe. If an MMPH tear is suspected from the preoperative MRI or

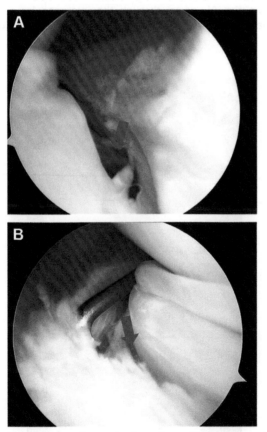

Fig. 2. (A) The longitudinal tear of posterior horn (*arrow*), seen from a 30° arthroscope, is inserted from the anterolateral portal to the posteromedial compartment. (B) The postero-medial portal and a probe verify the lesion.

during arthroscopic examination, or if ACL ligament was torn concomitantly, the posterior compartment is approached by passing the 30° arthroscope from AL portal through the intercondylar notch between the medial femoral condyle and the posterior cruciate ligament (PCL). This is first facilitated by placing the anterior portals close to the margins of the patellar tendon. Afterward, a standard PM portal is created under direct arthroscopic visualization. This makes instruments, such as the suture hook, easier to move and manipulate. Using a probe, the posterior compartment is examined thoroughly (**Fig. 2**).

Switching the scope to the PM portal, the posterior horn is re-examined. After establishing a suture plan, a 70° arthroscope is reinserted to the anterolateral portal and placed through the intercondylar notch to view the posterior compartment. The second PM portal, which is a superior PM portal, is marked 1 cm superior to the previous standard PM portal. The entry point is then localized with an 18-gauge spinal needle while viewing from inside. After the proper position is confirmed, a skin incision and subcutaneous dissection are performed. A 5.5-mm diameter universal cannula (Linvatec, Largo, FL, USA) is placed into this superior PM portal (**Fig. 3**).

All-inside meniscal suture technique using 2 posteromedial portals

While viewing from the AL portal through the intercondylar notch using a 70° arthroscope, a shaver or rasp is introduced through the PM portal without a cannula

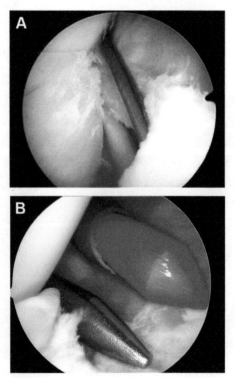

Fig. 3. (*A*) The tear pattern is clearly seen after changing to a 70° arthroscope, (*B*) The 2 posteromedial portals are established.

for debridement of both tear sides of the tear. A 45° curved suture hook (Linvatec) loaded with a polydioxanone synthetic (PDS) No. 0 (Ethicon, Somerville, NJ, USA) is inserted through the standard PM portal. The sharp hook tip first penetrates the meniscal peripheral rim tissue (meniscocapsular tissue) from superior to inferior. Then it is advanced under and across the tear before penetrating the mobile central fragment from inferior to superior. During this procedure, the surgeon must recognize that the peripheral rim of the torn meniscus is almost always displaced inferiorly relative to the mobile central fragment. Without caution, the entire thickness of the peripheral rim portion may not be penetrated, which will result in a poor tissue approximation. The surgeon can essentially verify this with the suture hook by penetrating the whole thickness of the peripheral rim and making the tip of the hook come out of the torn interval before making additional sutures at the mobile central fragment. Sometimes, the portion of the torn central meniscus may be difficult to pierce because of its mobility; in these situations, a probe can be inserted through the universal cannula to stabilize the inner fragment. The probe holds the central fragment down to the tibial surface, and the suture hook penetrates from the inferior to superior side. Using a suture retriever, both suture ends are brought out through the universal cannula. The SMC (Samsung Medical Center) knot[37] is tied and slid through the

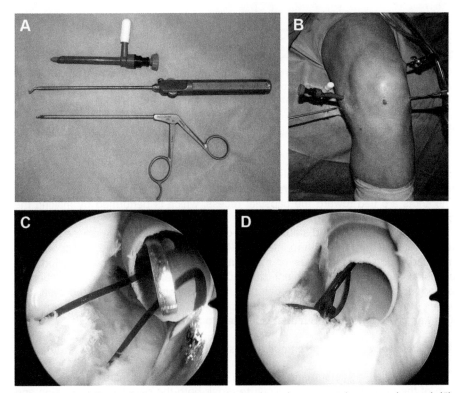

Fig. 4. (A) From above, the cannula, 45° suture hook, and suture retriever are observed. (B) During suturing, the arthroscope is placed in the anterolateral portal, the cannular is inserted to the superior posteromedial portal, and the suture hook is inserted into the posteromedial portal. (C) Both suture materials are held together and retrieved out of the posteromedial portal by the suture retriever through the cannula. (D) The sliding knot is used for knot tying.

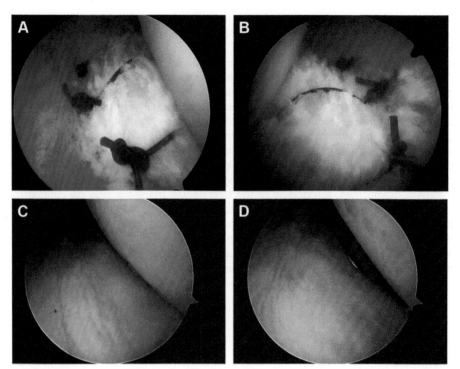

Fig. 5. (A) The 30° arthroscope inserted from posteromedial portal shows 3 vertical sutures at the longitudinal tear of posterior horn of medial meniscus. (B) The 70° arthroscope, inserted from anterolateral portal to the posteromedial compartment, shows the same findings. (C, D) Complete healing is shown on the second-look arthroscopy at 1 year, 9 months postoperatively.

cannula with a knot pusher. Additional 2 or 3 half-hitch knots with alternating posts on reverse throws are made, and the reduction is carefully inspected arthroscopically. The knots are tied toward the capsular recess, which is performed by making the capsular limb the post (**Fig. 4**).

For good coaptation and stable fixation of the torn meniscus, we advise placing 3 to 4 sutures with a 4- to 5-mm interval. If the tear is extended to the midbody, our modified inside-out technique or meniscal fixators are used in combination with all-inside suturing. If the patient has ACL insufficiency, ACL reconstruction is performed after the meniscal repair. For these patients, we repair the meniscus without tourniquet application and perform the ACL reconstruction with a tourniquet. This keeps the time the tourniquet is inflated to a minimum (**Fig. 5**).

All-inside meniscal suture technique using single posteromedial portal without cannula

This modified all-inside suturing technique is ideal for MMPH tears that are within 3 mm of the peripheral rim. It is difficult to repair both the peripheral rim portion and central fragment at once, in cases in which the MMPH is rather thick, which is typically seen with tears located within 3 to 5mm of the peripheral rim and double longitudinal tears within 5 mm of the peripheral rim. At this time, the shuttle relay system is used to repair from 2 times sutures to 1 suture (**Fig. 6**).

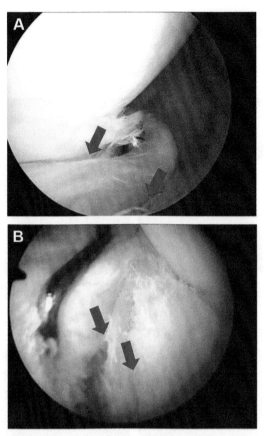

Fig. 6. (*A*) The 30° arthroscope inserted from posteromedial portal shows double longitudinal tears (*arrow*) at meniscocapsular junction of posterior horn of medial meniscus. (*B*) The 70° arthroscope, inserted from anterolateral portal to the posteromedial compartment, shows the same findings.

We suggest using a single PM portal without the use of a cannula for suture placement on the peripheral longitudinal tear of the MMPH. A suture hook loaded with PDS No. 0 is introduced to the PM portal, and then a suture passage is made starting from the inner tear penetrating the most central fragment from inferior to superior. During this procedure, care must be taken not to damage the cartilage of the femoral condyle, as the sharp tip of the hook passes close to the condyle during this procedure. Both ends of PDS No. 0 are taken out with a suture retriever through the PM portal. The superior end of the suture is marked with a straight hemostat, and the inferior suture end is left alone. A suture hook loaded with MAXON 2-0 (Syneture, Norwalk, CO, USA) is then inserted through the PM portal and used to penetrate the peripheral rim at the capsular side from the superior to inferior surface in the same manner. After both ends of MAXON are taken out of the PM portal with the suture retriever, the superior end of the suture is marked with a straight hemostat. The inferior side of the PDS and MAXON are held together and retrieved out of the PM portal using the suture retriever at the same time to avoid soft tissue interposition between both limbs. The inferior side end of MAXON 2-0 is then tied with the inferior side of the end of PDS, and the hemostat holding the superior end of MAXON is then pulled. The PDS is subsequently passed through both sides of the meniscal tear as the MAXON is changed for the PDS No.0 from the tibial to the femoral surface. Both ends of PDS are held together and retrieved at the same time

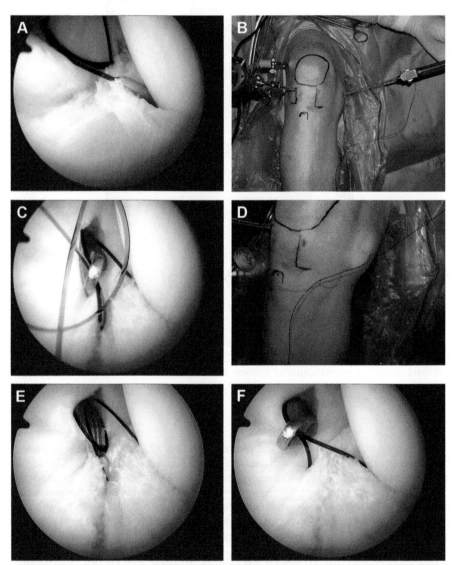

Fig. 7. (A) The 70° arthroscope, inserted from anterolateral portal to the posteromedial compartment, shows a suture passage is made starting from the inner tear penetrating the most central fragment from inferior to superior. (B) The outside picture shows these findings. (C) The inferior side of the PDS and MAXON are held together and retrieved out of the PM portal using the suture retriever at the same time. (D) The outside picture shows the MAXON is tied to the PDS for changing. (E) The PDS is subsequently passed through both sides of the meniscal tear as the MAXON is changed for the PDS from the tibial to the femoral surface. (F) Both ends of PDS are held together and retrieved at the same time through the posteromedial portal using a suture retriever.

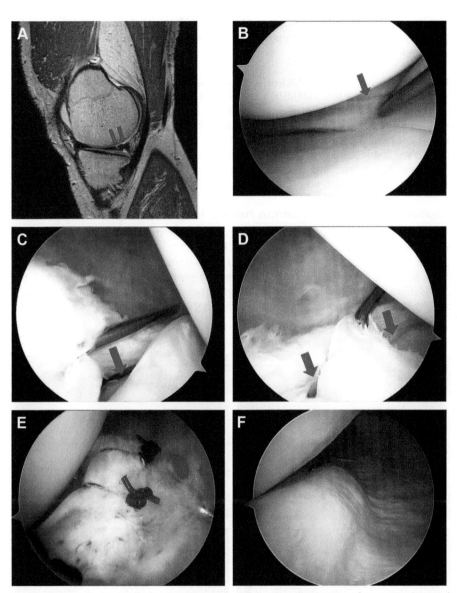

Fig. 8. (*A*) The sagittal MRI finding shows double longitudinal tears of posterior horn of medial meniscus (*arrow*). (*B*) The 30° arthroscope inserted from anterolateral portal shows longitudinal tear (*arrow*) of the posterior horn of the medial meniscus at the avascular area. (*C*) The 70° arthroscope, inserted from the anterolateral portal to the posteromedial compartment, shows longitudinal tear of posterior horn of medial meniscus at meniscocapsular junction area. (*D*) A partial meniscectomy (*arrow*) is performed on the avascular area. (*E*) The 30° arthroscope inserted from posteromedial portal shows the tear is repaired with vertical sutures at longitudinal tear of the posterior horn of medial meniscus around meniscocapsular junction. (*F*) Complete healing is shown on the second-look arthroscopy 2 years postoperatively.

through the PM portal using a suture retriever. A SMC knot is tied and slid through the cannula with a knot pusher, with additional securing half-hitch sutures. A firm repair is confirmed with a probe (**Fig. 7**).

All-inside meniscal suture technique in double longitudinal tear

A double longitudinal tear in MMPH is sometimes seen with chronic ACL insufficiency. To make the description simpler, between the 2 longitudinal tears, we named the more peripheral tear site as the outer tear and the more central tear site as the inner tear. If 2 longitudinal tears are located within 5 mm of the peripheral rim, all-inside sutures are used for the repair using a shuttle-relay system. If the inner tear is located more than 5 mm from the peripheral rim, the outer tear is repaired and a partial meniscectomy is performed on the inner tear (**Fig. 8**).

Longitudinal Tear of Lateral Meniscus Posterior Horn

Peripheral longitudinal tears of the lateral meniscus posterior horn (LMPH) are often associated with an ACL injury or discoid LM tear.[38-40] The LM is circular in shape, smaller in radius, thicker in periphery, and more mobile than the medial meniscus. Such anatomic characteristics may render the peripheral longitudinal tear of the LMPH more difficult to repair. In the anatomically more confined PL compartment, it is difficult to make 2 portals, and the working span of instruments is very limited. To

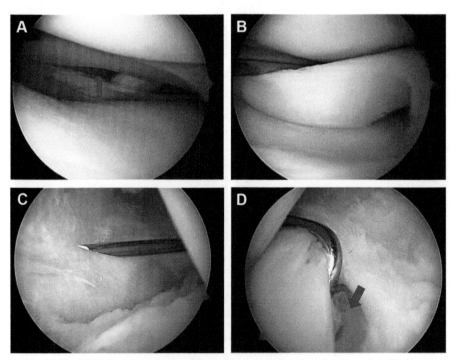

Fig. 9. (*A*) The 30° arthroscope inserted from the anterolateral portal shows longitudinal tear (*arrow*) of the posterior horn of the lateral meniscus. (*B*) The tear is seen unstable and displaceable with a probe. (*C*) A posterolateral portal is created under direct arthroscopic visualization. (*D*) The 30° arthroscope inserted from posterolateral portal shows the longitudinal tear (*arrow*) of the posterior horn of the lateral meniscus around the meniscocapsular junction.

amend such limitations, we introduce the arthroscopic all-inside suture of LMPH tear by a single PL portal.[24] Our suturing technique allows greater freedom in suture hook maneuvering by using a single PL portal without a cannula. This technique allows excellent visualization of the PL compartment, anatomic coaptation of the torn meniscus, and strong knot tying, while avoiding inadvertent injury to the remnant meniscus and articular cartilage. In patients with a discoid LM, we sometimes found a tear at the posterior horn or a meniscocapsular junction separation from the popliteal hiatus to the posterior horn after performing a central meniscectomy.[38,39] Because such lesions dispose the LMPH to instability, they should be repaired. We suggest using a single standard PL portal without the use of a cannula for suture placement on the peripheral longitudinal tear of the LMPH.

Diagnostic arthroscopy

A diagnostic arthroscopic examination of the knee is performed using the standard AL and AM portals. For easy access to the PL compartment, the AM portal should be placed just medial to the patella tendon, right above the MM. With discoid lateral menisci, it is often difficult to find the peripheral longitudinal tear at the posterior horn through a standard anterior portal because the thick meniscal tissue may obstruct the

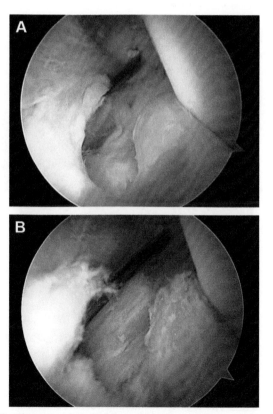

Fig. 10. (*A*) The 70° arthroscope inserted from the anteromedial portal to the posterolateral compartment, shows the longitudinal tear of posterior horn of lateral meniscus. (*B*) A shaver or rasp is introduced through the posterolateral portal without a cannula for debridement of both tear sides of the tear.

visualization of a posterior horn tear. The PL compartment can be approached by passing a 30° arthroscope between the anterior cruciate ligament and the lateral femoral condyle. Once a peripheral longitudinal tear of the LMPH horn is confirmed with standard diagnostic arthroscopy, the 70° arthroscope can be used for better visualization. Various anatomic structures in the PL compartment, such as the LMPH, the PL capsules, and the lateral femoral condyle are examined using a 30° arthroscope inserted at the AM portal and passed through the intercondylar notch. While keeping the knee flexed at 90° for maximal joint distension and to avoid neurovascular injury, an 18-gauge spinal needle is inserted at the PL corner under transillumination. After making a stab skin incision, followed by widening with a hemostat, a probe is inserted to examine the extent, degree, and shape of the peripheral tear at the LMPH. A switching stick is inserted to keep the PL portal open. The arthroscope is then inserted over the switching stick to examine the PL compartment and the torn LMPH from a different view (**Fig. 9**).

Repairing a peripheral longitudinal tear of the lateral meniscus posterior horn

While viewing from the AM portal through the intercondylar notch using a 70° arthroscope, a shaver or rasp is introduced through the PL portal for debridement of

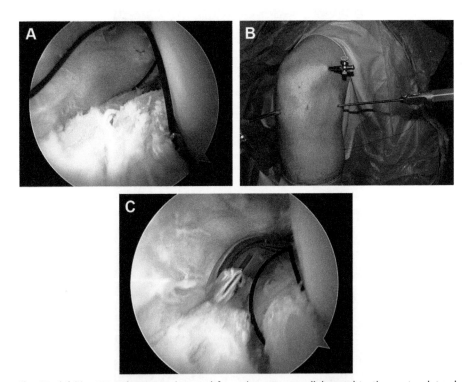

Fig. 11. (*A*) The 70° arthroscope, inserted from the anteromedial portal to the posterolateral compartment, shows a suture passage is made starting from the inner tear penetrating the most central fragment from inferior to superior. (*B*) The outside picture shows these findings. (*C*) The suture hook loaded with MAXON is inserted through the posterolateral portal and used to penetrate the peripheral rim at the capsular side from the superior to inferior surface in the same manner.

both tear sites. The 70° arthroscope is typically used for better visualization. Inserting and manipulating instruments without a cannula allows more freedom to use the instrument in the relatively restricted PL compartment (**Fig. 10**).

After preparation of the tear site, a 45° angled suture hook loaded with PDS No. 0 is introduced to the PL portal, and then a suture is made starting from the inner tear penetrating the most central fragment from inferior to superior direction. Once again, care must be taken not to damage the cartilage of the femoral condyle. Both ends of PDS No. 0 are taken out with suture retriever through the PL portal. The superior end of the suture is marked with a straight hemostat, and the inferior suture end is left alone. The suture hook loaded with MAXON 2-0 is inserted through the PL portal and used to penetrate the peripheral rim at the capsular side from the superior to inferior surface in the same manner (**Fig. 11**).

After both ends of MAXON are taken out with a suture retriever through the PL portal, the superior end of the suture is marked with a straight hemostat. The inferior side of the PDS and MAXON are held together and retrieved out of the PL portal using the suture retriever at the same time to avoid soft tissue interposition between both ends. And then, the inferior side end of MAXON 2-0 is tied to the inferior side of the end of PDS, and the hemostat holding superior end of MAXON is then pulled. The

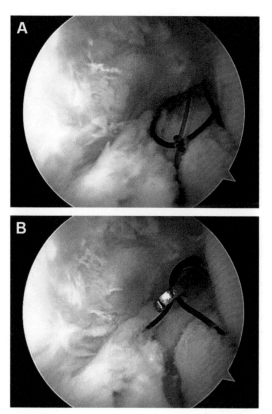

Fig. 12. (*A*) The PDS is subsequently passed through both sides of the meniscal tear as the MAXON is changed for the PDS No.0 from the tibial to the femoral surface. (*B*) Both ends of PDS are held together and retrieved at the same time through the posterolateral portal using a suture retriever.

PDS is passed across sides of the meniscal tear as the MAXON is pulled. Both ends of PDS are held together and retrieved through the PL portal. The SMC knot is tied and used to secure the repair (**Fig. 12**).

Depending on the size of a tear, additional sutures can be made. Usually 2 to 3 sutures are adequate for the repair of the longitudinal tear on the LMPH. If an ACL tear is required, it is performed subsequent to the meniscus repair (**Fig. 13**).

Radial Tears of Midbody or Root of the Lateral Meniscus

Meniscus functions are maintained by mostly circumferential fibers of the collagen bundles of the meniscus.[18,41–43] Therefore, radial tears of the meniscus are more biomechanically detrimental than longitudinal tears.[44] However, most radial tears are treated by partial meniscectomy. Meniscal repair may be an alternative treatment for radial tears involving the red-red or red-white zone to preserve the important functions of the meniscus (**Fig. 14**).[45,46]

Diagnostic arthroscopy

A diagnostic arthroscopic examination of the knee is performed using the standard AL and AM portals. While viewing with arthroscopy through the AM portal, the tear site is

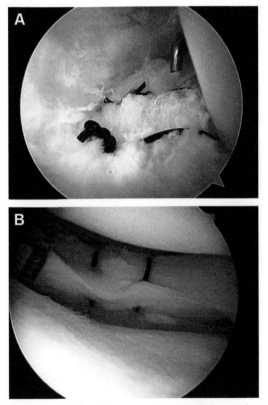

Fig. 13. (*A*) The 70° arthroscope, inserted from anteromedial portal to the posterolateral compartment, shows 2 vertical sutures at the longitudinal tear of the posterior horn of lateral meniscus. (*B*) The 30° arthroscope, inserted from anterolateral portal, also shows anatomic coaptation of the lateral meniscus posterior horn tear with 2 vertical sutures.

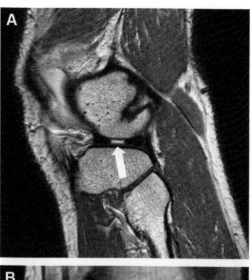

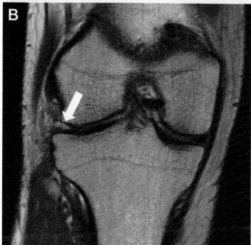

Fig. 14. (*A*) The sagittal MRI finding shows cutoff of the margin in midbody of the lateral meniscus (*arrow*). (*B*) The coronal MRI finding shows disappearance of midbody of the lateral meniscus (*arrow*).

evaluated with probe inserted through AL portal with the knee in a "figure-4" position. Arthroscopic examination confirms a radial tear of the midbody of the LM involving the red-red or red-white zone of the LM (**Fig. 15**).

Repairing for radial tear of the midbody of the lateral meniscus

Gentle debridement is performed at the tear site using a motorized shaver. A vertical suture can be inserted in top-to-bottom fashion or vice versa, according to which approach is more feasible. A straight suture hook loaded with PDS No. 0 is introduced through the AL portal and then penetrates the anterior part of the LM from a superior to inferior direction. Both ends of PDS No. 0 are taken out with suture retriever through the AL portal. The superior end of the suture is marked with a straight

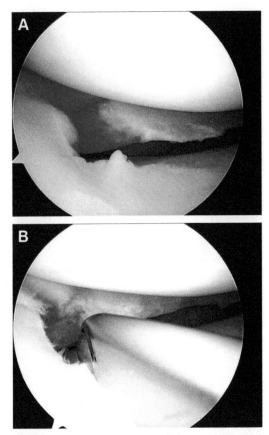

Fig. 15. (*A*) The arthroscope shows the extended radial tear to the meniscocapsular junction in midbody of the lateral meniscus. (*B*) A shaver is introduced for debridement of both tear sides of the tear.

hemostat, and the inferior suture end is left alone. The suture hook loaded with MAXON 2-0 is inserted through the AL portal and used to penetrate the posterior part of the LM in the same manner (**Fig. 16**).

The bottom side of the PDS and MAXON are held together and retrieved out of the AL portal using the suture retriever at the same time to avoid soft tissue interposition between both ends. As before, the bottom end of MAXON 2-0 is tied with the bottom end of the PDS. The hemostat holding the superior end of MAXON is then pulled bringing the PDS suture across the tear from the tibial to femoral surface. Both ends of PDS are retrieved through the AL portal and tied using a SMC sliding knot. One or 2 sutures are placed according to the tear length and approximation (**Fig. 17**).

The LM root tears are defined as radial tears located within 1 cm of the posterior horn bony attachment. About 7% of patients undergoing ACL reconstructions had concomitant LM root tears. Double attachments of the root are observed in the posterior horn of the LM, with the anterior portion attached to the tibial intercondylar eminence and the posterior portion to the femoral medial condyle through the meniscofemoral ligaments. Therefore, the possibility exists that displaced posterior LM root tears may be overlooked as a posterior-based flap tear even if the bony

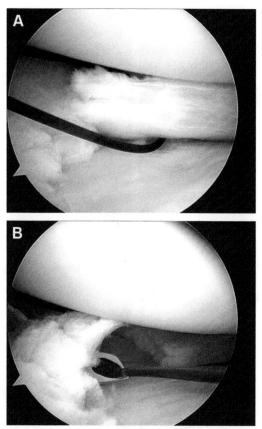

Fig. 16. (*A*) The 30° arthroscope, inserted from the anteromedial portal, shows a suture passage is made at the posterior side. (*B*) The suture hook loaded with MAXON is inserted through the anterior side from the superior to inferior surface.

attachment has been completely transected (**Fig. 18**). The confusion between a complete radial tear and a flap tear of the posterior root likely occurs because of a residual meniscofemoral attachment. In this situation, partial meniscectomy of the torn portion of the meniscus may lead to poor clinical results because of loss of the meniscus' hoop stress. To restore the meniscus' hoop stress, the LM root tears should be repaired with same surgical technique as that of midbody repair before ACL reconstruction (**Fig. 19**).[40,47]

POSTOPERATIVE CARE

The protocol for postoperative rehabilitation follows guidelines similar to those advocated for rehabilitation of ACL reconstruction. The knee is immobilized in a full extension in a brace for 2 weeks. Gradual range of motion is initiated with a limited-motion brace, in which at least 90° of flexion is achieved during the 4- and 6-week postoperative period. Crutches are used full time for the first 4 weeks postoperatively to protect the repair site. Patients are allowed to begin full weight bearing by the fourth postoperative week. Squatting, or deep flexion, greater than

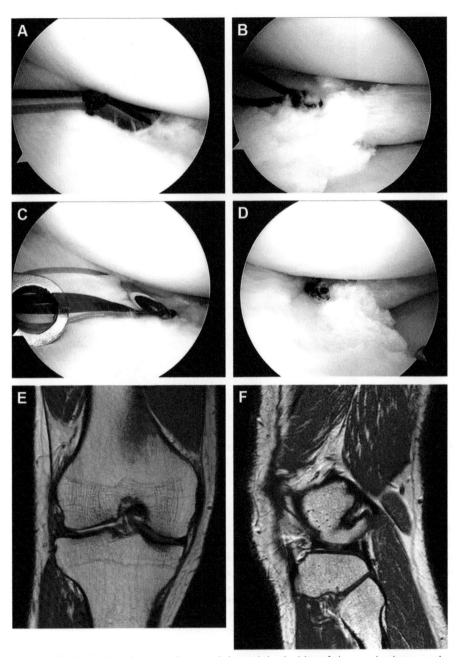

Fig. 17. (*A*) The PDS is subsequently passed through both sides of the meniscal tear as the MAXON is changed for the PDS. (*B*) The sliding knot is used for knot tying. (*C*) Both ends of PDS are held together and retrieved to the MAXON loop using a suture retriever. (*D*) The vertical suture is seen at the radial tear of midbody of the lateral meniscus. (*E, F*) The coronal and sagittal MRI findings show healing process in radial tear of the lateral meniscus midbody 5 months postoperatively.

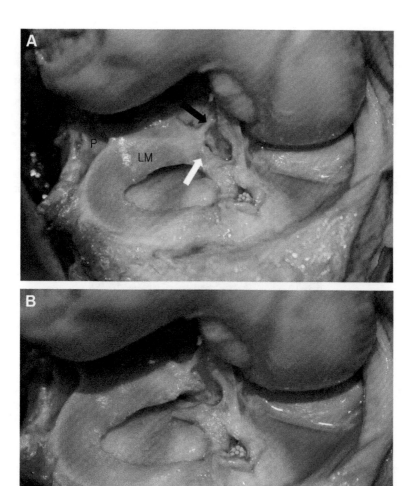

Fig. 18. (*A*) Images of a disarticulated knee with the femur removed looking down on the menisci show 2 insertions. (*black arrow*, insertion to meniscofemoral ligament; *white arrow*, insertion to bone) (*B*) After the tear of bony insertion, only insertion to meniscofemoral ligament remained and the lateral meniscus was subluxed posteriorly.

120°, is restricted for at least 8 weeks. Patients are told to avoid sports that require jumping, cutting, or twisting maneuvers for 6 months.

AUTHORS' CLINICAL OUTCOMES

We evaluated 140 patients who underwent MMPH repair using either a modified all-inside or inside-out technique with concomitant ACL reconstruction performed by a second-look arthroscopy at a mean of 37.7 months postoperatively.[40] Among 140 patients, 118 (84.3%) showed complete healing, 17 (12.1%) had incomplete healing, and 5 (3.6%) did not heal. The clinical success rate was 96.4% (135 of 140) because

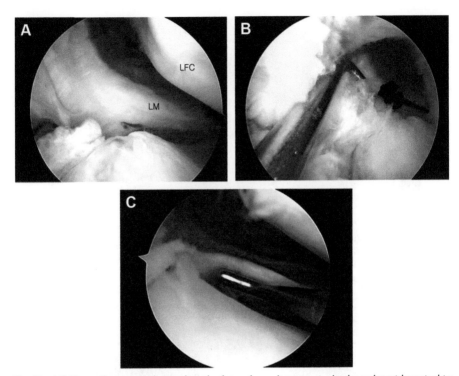

Fig. 19. (*A*) The arthroscope shows that the lateral meniscus posterior horn is not inserted to the bone. (*B*) The remaining meniscus is repaired to the flap of bony insertion. (*C*) Completely healed meniscus with nearly normal hoop tension is confirmed 2 years postoperatively.

patients in the incomplete group showed no clinical symptoms associated with meniscal tears.

We also reported on 23 children (28 knees) with peripheral tear in symptomatic discoid LM that was treated by partial central meniscectomy in conjunction with peripheral suture repair.[39] Arthroscopic findings were categorized into 3 types in terms of peripheral rim stability and tear site: (1) meniscocapsular junction, anterior horn type; (2) meniscocapsular junction, posterior horn type; and (3) posterolateral corner loss type. These 3 types needed different arthroscopic techniques for saucerization with repair. All patients were able to return to their previous life activities with little or no limitation, and no reoperation was required after an average follow-up of 51 months.

REFERENCES

1. Arnoczky SP, Warren RF. Microvasculature of the human meniscus. Am J Sports Med 1982;10:90–5.
2. Arnoczky SP, Warren RF. The microvasculature of the meniscus and its response to injury. An experimental study in the dog. Am J Sports Med 1983;11:131–41.
3. Ahn JH, Wang JH, Oh I. Modified inside-out technique for meniscal repair. Arthroscopy 2004;20(Suppl 2):178–82.
4. Brown GC, Rosenberg TD, Deffner KT. Inside-out meniscal repair using zone-specific instruments. Am J Knee Surg 1996;9:144–50.

5. Cannon WD Jr. Arthroscopic meniscal repair. Inside-out technique and results. Am J Knee Surg 1996;9:137–43.
6. Horibe S, Shino K, Nakata K, et al. Second-look arthroscopy after meniscal repair. Review of 132 menisci repaired by an arthroscopic inside-out technique. J Bone Joint Surg Br 1995;77:245–9.
7. Austin KS, Sherman OH. Complications of arthroscopic meniscal repair. Am J Sports Med 1993;21:864–8[discussion: 8–9].
8. Small NC. Complications in arthroscopic surgery performed by experienced arthroscopists. Arthroscopy 1988;4:215–21.
9. Barber FA, Coons DA. Midterm results of meniscal repair using the BioStinger meniscal repair device. Arthroscopy 2006;22:400–5.
10. Kotsovolos ES, Hantes ME, Mastrokalos DS, et al. Results of all-inside meniscal repair with the FasT-Fix meniscal repair system. Arthroscopy 2006;22:3–9.
11. Koukoulias N, Papastergiou S, Kazakos K, et al. Clinical results of meniscus repair with the meniscus arrow: a 4- to 8-year follow-up study. Knee Surg Sports Traumatol Arthrosc 2007;15:133–7.
12. Quinby JS, Golish SR, Hart JA, et al. All-inside meniscal repair using a new flexible, tensionable device. Am J Sports Med 2006;34:1281–6.
13. Anderson K, Marx RG, Hannafin J, et al. Chondral injury following meniscal repair with a biodegradable implant. Arthroscopy 2000;16:749–53.
14. Dervin GF, Downing KJ, Keene GC, et al. Failure strengths of suture versus biodegradable arrow for meniscal repair: an in vitro study. Arthroscopy 1997;13:296–300.
15. Song EK, Lee KB, Yoon TR. Aseptic synovitis after meniscal repair using the biodegradable meniscus arrow. Arthroscopy 2001;17:77–80.
16. Nakamae A, Deie M, Yasumoto M, et al. Synovial cyst formation resulting from nonabsorbable meniscal repair devices for meniscal repair. Arthroscopy 2004;20 (Suppl 2):16–9.
17. Cohen SB, Boyd L, Miller MD. Vascular risk associated with meniscal repair using Rapidloc versus FasT-Fix: comparison of two all-inside meniscal devices. J Knee Surg 2007;20:235–40.
18. Hospodar SJ, Schmitz MR, Golish SR, et al. FasT-Fix versus inside-out suture meniscal repair in the goat model. Am J Sports Med 2009;37:330–3.
19. Miller MD, Kline AJ, Jepsen KG. "All-inside" meniscal repair devices: an experimental study in the goat model. Am J Sports Med 2004;32:858–62.
20. Morgan CD. The "all-inside" meniscus repair. Arthroscopy 1991;7:120–5.
21. Rimmer MG, Nawana NS, Keene GC, et al. Failure strengths of different meniscal suturing techniques. Arthroscopy 1995;11:146–50.
22. Ahn JH, Kim SH, Yoo JC, et al. All-inside suture technique using two posteromedial portals in a medial meniscus posterior horn tear. Arthroscopy 2004;20:101–8.
23. Ahn JH, Wang JH, Yoo JC. Arthroscopic all-inside suture repair of medial meniscus lesion in anterior cruciate ligament–deficient knees: results of second-look arthroscopies in 39 cases. Arthroscopy 2004;20:936–45.
24. Ahn JH, Oh I. Arthroscopic all-inside lateral meniscus suture using posterolateral portal. Arthroscopy 2006;22:572, e1–4.
25. Indelicato PA, Bittar ES. A perspective of lesions associated with ACL insufficiency of the knee. A review of 100 cases. Clin Orthop Relat Res 1985:77–80.
26. Noyes FR, Barber-Westin SD. Arthroscopic repair of meniscus tears extending into the avascular zone with or without anterior cruciate ligament reconstruction in patients 40 years of age and older. Arthroscopy 2000;16:822–9.
27. Henning CE. Current status of meniscus salvage. Clin Sports Med 1990;9:567–76.

28. Warren RF, Marshall JL. Injuries of the anterior cruciate and medial collateral ligaments of the knee. A long-term follow-up of 86 cases—part II. Clin Orthop Relat Res 1978:198–211.

29. Yoo JC, Ahn JH, Lee SH, et al. Increasing incidence of medial meniscal tears in nonoperatively treated anterior cruciate ligament insufficiency patients documented by serial magnetic resonance imaging studies. Am J Sports Med 2009;37:1478–83.

30. Levy IM, Torzilli PA, Warren RF. The effect of medial meniscectomy on anterior-posterior motion of the knee. J Bone Joint Surg Am 1982;64:883–8.

31. Ahn JH, Lee YS, Yoo JC, et al. Clinical and second-look arthroscopic evaluation of repaired medial meniscus in anterior cruciate ligament-reconstructed knees. Am J Sports Med 2010;38:472–7.

32. Pujol N, Beaufils P. Healing results of meniscal tears left in situ during anterior cruciate ligament reconstruction: a review of clinical studies. Knee Surg Sports Traumatol Arthrosc 2009;17:396–401.

33. Yagishita K, Muneta T, Ogiuchi T, et al. Healing potential of meniscal tears without repair in knees with anterior cruciate ligament reconstruction. Am J Sports Med 2004;32:1953–61.

34. De Smet AA, Graf BK. Meniscal tears missed on MR imaging: relationship to meniscal tear patterns and anterior cruciate ligament tears. AJR Am J Roentgenol 1994;162:905–11.

35. Rubin DA, Britton CA, Towers JD, et al. Are MR imaging signs of meniscocapsular separation valid? Radiology 1996;201:829–36.

36. Sanchis-Alfonso V, Martinez-Sanjuan V, Gastaldi-Orquin E. The value of MRI in the evaluation of the ACL deficient knee and in the post-operative evaluation after ACL reconstruction. Eur J Radiol 1993;16:126–30.

37. Kim SH, Ha KI. The SMC knot—a new slip knot with locking mechanism. Arthroscopy 2000;16:563–5.

38. Ahn JH, Choi SH, Lee YS, et al. Symptomatic torn discoid lateral meniscus in adults. Knee Surg Sports Traumatol Arthrosc 2011;19:158–64.

39. Ahn JH, Lee SH, Yoo JC, et al. Arthroscopic partial meniscectomy with repair of the peripheral tear for symptomatic discoid lateral meniscus in children: results of minimum 2 years of follow-up. Arthroscopy 2008;24:888–98.

40. Ahn JH, Lee YS, Yoo JC, et al. Results of arthroscopic all-inside repair for lateral meniscus root tear in patients undergoing concomitant anterior cruciate ligament reconstruction. Arthroscopy 2010;26:67–75.

41. Voloshin AS, Wosk J. Shock absorption of meniscectomized and painful knees: a comparative in vivo study. J Biomed Eng 1983;5:157–61.

42. Walker PS, Erkman MJ. The role of the menisci in force transmission across the knee. Clin Orthop Relat Res 1975:184–92.

43. Wojtys EM, Chan DB. Meniscus structure and function. Instr Course Lect 2005;54:323–30.

44. Harper KW, Helms CA, Lambert HS 3rd, et al. Radial meniscal tears: significance, incidence, and MR appearance. AJR Am J Roentgenol 2005;185:1429–34.

45. Choi NH, Kim TH, Son KM, et al. Meniscal repair for radial tears of the midbody of the lateral meniscus. Am J Sports Med 2010;38:2472–6.

46. Yoo JC, Ahn JH, Lee SH, et al. Suturing complete radial tears of the lateral meniscus. Arthroscopy 2007;23:1249, e1–7.

47. Ahn JH, Lee YS, Chang JY, et al. Arthroscopic all inside repair of the lateral meniscus root tear. Knee 2009;16:77–80.

Meniscus Repair in Children

Cordelia W. Carter, MD, Mininder S. Kocher, MD, MPH*

KEYWORDS

- Child • Adolescent • Athlete • Knee injury • Meniscus
- Discoid

Once considered rare, meniscal injuries in children and adolescents are now widely recognized as a significant source of pain and dysfunction in the young person. The rise in the incidence of meniscal injury in youth is likely a combination of increasing recognition of the problem—aided by improved diagnostic imaging techniques such as magnetic resonance imaging (MRI)—as well as a true increase in the number of intra-articular knee injuries. Indeed, as the international trend towards earlier participation in organized sports at higher levels of competition continues to evolve, a corresponding increase in the number of sports-related injuries sustained in children and adolescents has been noted. In one study performed by the National Center for Injury Prevention and Control during the years 1997-1999, the rate of sports-related injury in persons aged 5-24 years was estimated to be nearly 60 injury episodes per 1000 persons annually.[1] Of these, injuries to the lower extremity were the most common. Happily, most sports-related injuries are minor and self-limited in nature—these include bruises, lacerations, and muscular strains. However, some injuries may be associated with significant short- and long-term morbidity and it is imperative that these be recognized and appropriately treated. Acute hemarthrosis of the knee in a young person, for example, is almost always abnormal and indicative of significant underlying pathology.[2,3] To better understand the types and frequency of intra-articular injuries associated with acute traumatic hemarthrosis of the knee, one group of authors performed diagnostic knee arthroscopy of 70 consecutive patients aged 7 to 18 years who presented with an acutely swollen knee following an injury. They reported that, for patients aged 7-12 years (preadolescents), meniscal injury was present 53% of the time and injury of the anterior cruciate ligament (ACL) was present 53% of the time. Six percent of preadolescents had a combined injury pattern (concomitant meniscus tear and ACL tear). For adolescents aged 13 to 18 years, meniscal injury was present in 45% of the knees and ACL injury in 73%, with 18% of these patients having a combined injury pattern. Importantly, nearly 75% of all

The authors did not receive funding in support of this manuscript.

The authors have nothing to disclose.

Division of Sports Medicine, Children's Hospital Boston, 300 Longwood Avenue, Boston, MA 02115, USA

* Corresponding author.

E-mail address: mininder.kocher@childrens.harvard.edu

doi:10.1016/j.csm.2011.09.002
0278-5919/12/$ – see front matter © 2012 Elsevier Inc. All rights reserved.

knee injuries in this series were sustained during sports participation.[2] With an unprecedented number of children and adolescents currently participating in sports and the relatively high rates of injury sustained during athletic participation, it is clear that meniscal injuries do occur in this population with some frequency. We know additionally that meniscal injuries are often associated with hemarthrosis of the knee, they are frequently sports related, and they commonly occur in the setting of concomitant intra-articular pathology, such as ACL tear. As a result, the appropriate diagnosis and timely management of meniscal tears in children and adolescents are crucial for optimizing long-term knee function in the young athlete.

BACKGROUND
Gross Anatomy

The menisci are C-shaped wedges of fibrocartilage located in the medial and lateral compartments of the knee.[4] They are formed early in fetal life and it has been demonstrated that by 14 weeks' gestational age, the medial and lateral menisci have assumed their characteristic appearances and anatomic relationships within the developing knee joint.[5] Specifically, the medial meniscus is semicircular in shape and is firmly anchored within the knee by its attachments to the intercondylar fossa, the joint capsule, and the deep fibers of the medial collateral ligament (MCL). By contrast, the lateral meniscus is more circular and covers a higher proportion (70%) of the lateral tibial plateau. It is stabilized within the joint by attachments to the intercondylar fossa and joint capsule via the variable meniscofemoral ligaments of Humphrey and Wrisberg. Unlike the medial meniscus, the lateral meniscus does not have an attachment to its adjacent collateral ligament; furthermore, in the area of the popliteal hiatus, the lateral meniscus is devoid entirely of peripheral capsular attachments. These factors render the lateral meniscus more mobile than the medial meniscus, and it is able to be translated 9 to 11 mm onto the tibia during normal knee motion.[4]

Biochemistry

The menisci are composed of a combination of molecules, including collagen, water, elastin, proteoglycans, and fibrochondrocytes. The collagen found in the menisci is primarily Type I collagen, which represents up to 70% of the meniscal dry weight.[4] These collagen fibers are arranged into a highly organized ultrastructure, with the deeper layer of circumferentially arranged fibers providing the majority of tensile strength to the meniscus. Radial, oblique, and vertically oriented collagen fibers aid in resisting hoop stresses.[6,7] Additionally, mechanoreceptors and Type I and II sensory fibers are also present in the meniscus and are believed to provide proprioceptive feedback for the knee.[4]

Function

The menisci play an important role in preservation of the articular cartilage through a combination of load sharing and shock absorption capabilities; specifically, the unique orientation of the collagen fibers in the menisci enables them to dissipate compressive loads placed across the knee joint. This important role as "shock absorber" was elucidated nicely by early biomechanical studies such as that published by Ahmed and colleagues in 1983. These authors investigated the contact pressures in the medial compartment of the knee prior to and following medial meniscectomy. Working with cadaver knees in the laboratory, they were able to demonstrate a significant decrease in the contact area in the medial compartment of 50% to 70% following total meniscectomy. Importantly, the postmeniscectomy reduction in contact area was associated with increases in both local peak pressures and high-pressure areas within the knee.[8]

Taking it a step further, Baratz and coworkers investigated the biomechanical effects of meniscal repair on contact pressures in the knee. Working with cadaver knees in the laboratory, these authors reproduced earlier findings by demonstrating significant increases in contact pressures following meniscectomy (on average, they reported greater than 200% increase in peak local contact stresses following total meniscectomy). Even more interesting, they found that creating peripheral meniscal tears and then repairing them through either open or closed means returned the peak pressure to near baseline levels.[9] From these findings, it can be extrapolated that meniscal integrity is of paramount importance in ameliorating contact pressures within the knee, which in turn protects the articular cartilage from injury and degeneration. This assumption has robust support in the literature: numerous authors have investigated the long-term effects of meniscectomy on the knee joint, with the majority reporting early degenerative changes on radiographs, lower clinical function scores, and increased subjective patient report of knee pain in postmeniscectomy patients.[10–20]

Blood Supply

As a result of these findings, meniscal preservation has become a primary focus in the treatment of children and adolescents. One important difference in this younger patient population is the meniscal blood supply. Cadaveric studies of the development of the human meniscus prenatally and postnatally have demonstrated that the meniscus begins as a highly cellular, fully vascularized structure, with a primary blood supply stemming from the medial and lateral geniculate arteries. These blood vessels arborize and form a circumferential capillary plexus that provides vascularity to the meniscus from its periphery.[5,7] Over the course of development, the vascularity of the meniscus gradually recedes, and by the age of 9 months, its inner third is relatively avascular. This trend continues over the first 10 years of life, with a gradual attrition of the blood supply to the central aspect of the meniscus. By the time adulthood is reached, there is a distinct lack of both vascularity and cellularity in the meniscus, with the exception of its peripheral 10% to 30%.[5,21] This has led some authors to demarcate the meniscus into 3 zones based on vascularity: the well-vascularized outer 3 mm is termed the "red-red" zone, the middle 3 to 5 millimeters is the "red-white" zone, and the most central meniscal tissue (rim width >5 mm) is termed the "white-white" zone.[21] In preadolescents and adolescents, however, the blood supply to the meniscus is highly variable. Regions in the central two-thirds of the meniscus that are avascular in the mature adult knee may in fact still be well-vascularized in this population. Due to this relatively increased meniscal vascularity, it is theorized that meniscal tears in younger patients are more likely to heal than those in adults.

Meniscal Healing

The pattern of vascularity is highly relevant to any discussion of meniscal injury, because there is good evidence that avascular regions of the meniscus are unable to undergo a significant reparative response to injury. As early as 1936, King reported his observations on the healing potential of meniscal injuries in dogs. This author surgically created a variety of meniscal tears in 13 healthy dogs and then reexamined them following death 2 to 14 weeks later. He noted that meniscal tears that were in continuity with the peripheral synovium were able to heal effectively, while those tears that were "limited to the semilunar cartilage" were not.[22] Nearly 50 years later,

Arnoczky and Warren expanded upon this work, surgically creating both transverse and longitudinal meniscal tears in laboratory dogs. At the time of death 10 weeks later, these authors noted that the meniscal tears that communicated with the peripheral blood supply had healed with a fibrovascular scar, while the longitudinal tears in the avascular central area of the meniscus had not. They additionally found that longitudinal tears of the meniscus that communicated with the periphery via "vascular access channels" were able to demonstrate a healing response. They concluded that the "blood supply appears sufficient to effect a reparative process in those meniscal lesions with which it communicates."[21] In other words, meniscal tears with an adequate vascular supply are more likely to heal than those without, and factors that maximize the blood supply to a torn meniscus—younger age, peripheral location, vascular "channels"—will therefore optimize its healing potential.

MENISCAL INJURIES
Traumatic Meniscal Tears

Background
Traumatic meniscal injuries in the pediatric and adolescent population are most frequently the result of a noncontact, twisting injury to the knee. They are very frequently sports-related. Traumatic meniscal injuries generally occur in older children and adolescents although there have been case reports of traumatic meniscal tears requiring surgical repair in patients as young as 4 years of age.[23] Young patients with a meniscal tear will usually cite knee pain as their primary complaint. Knee swelling and mechanical knee symptoms such as; snapping, giving way, locking, or catching may also be reported. Unlike older children and adults, who are generally able to give a thorough history of injury and comply with a targeted physical examination, younger children may be unable to clearly recall and recount the episode of injury or to tolerate manipulation of the painful knee. Because children may be unable or unwilling to cooperate with the physician, physical examination in this patient population may be particularly tricky. That said the presence of a joint effusion with associated joint line tenderness is highly suggestive of meniscal pathology and should be sought and noted. Range of motion should be evaluated and compared with the unaffected contralateral knee, as loss of motion may be a subtle sign of meniscal pathology. Provocative maneuvers such as the McMurray's test, if tolerated by the patient, are also associated with meniscal tear and may be helpful in making the diagnosis. Finally, because of the high rate of associated intra-articular pathology associated with meniscal tear, a thorough examination of the ligamentous structures of the knee (Lachman testing, anterior and posterior drawer testing, varus and valgus stress tests, dial testing) should also be routinely performed. As alluded to earlier, examination of both knees is imperative. Interestingly, a recent study noted that the sensitivity and specificity of the clinical examination for detecting meniscal tears were 50% and 89% for the lateral meniscus and 62% and 81% for the medial meniscus, respectively. Additionally, the negative predictive value of clinical examination for meniscal injuries was extremely high (94% and 98% for the lateral and medial meniscus, respectively).[24]

Differential diagnosis for meniscal tear in the preadolescent and adolescent patient includes ACL tear; tibial eminence fracture; osteochondritis dissecans (OCD) lesions of the femur, tibia, or patella; pathologic plica; patellar instability; osteochondral fracture; intra-articular loose body; and chondral flap tears.

Diagnostic imaging of the acutely injured knee typically includes 4 radiographic views—anteroposterior, lateral, notch, and skyline. These enable the clinician to evaluate for osseous abnormalities such as fractures, loose bodies, and OCD lesions. In the setting of isolated meniscal injury, however, radiographs are frequently normal and the use of adjunctive diagnostic imaging (MRI) has become increasingly common. According to a recent study by Kocher and colleagues, who investigated the ability of MRI and clinical examination to diagnose intra-articular disorders of the knee in the pediatric population, MRI has a sensitivity of 67% and 79%, respectively, for the diagnosis of lateral and medial meniscal tears in children. The specificity of MRI for the diagnosis of medial meniscal tear is 92%, which is significantly greater than that for clinical examination alone.[24] That said, MRI should not take the place of a thorough physical examination: there is good evidence that MRI in the pediatric population is less sensitive and specific in younger children (<12 years old) than it is in older children and adolescents. Additionally, the increased vascularity of the normal meniscus in younger children may mimic tearing of the meniscus, leading to a high false-positive rate in this population.[24]

Treatment

Indications for nonoperative treatment of traumatic meniscal tears in children are few. Examples of meniscal tears that are amenable to nonoperative intervention include partial thickness tears (involving <50% of the meniscal thickness); small tears (<10 mm); and stable, longitudinal tears in the peripheral red-red zone (<3 mm from the meniscosynovial junction). This type of meniscal tear is usually found at the time of diagnostic arthroscopy performed in the setting of ACL reconstruction and has an excellent chance of healing spontaneously. When found in isolation, these small, peripheral tears may be treated with protected motion and weightbearing in a hinged knee brace for 4 weeks, with supervised physical therapy and gradual return to cutting and pivoting sports at 12 weeks postinjury.

Most meniscal tears will require surgical intervention, and for these, diagnostic arthroscopy with thorough evaluation of the tear is the standard first step. The meniscal tear must be thoroughly evaluated. Visual inspection of the tear elicits information about its location, rim width, size and configuration (longitudinal, oblique, radial, horizontal, or complex). Palpation of the tear with an arthroscopic probe enables the surgeon to directly evaluate the quality of the meniscal tissue and the stability of the tear. Inspection of the entire joint should be performed at the time of diagnostic arthroscopy to ensure that all associated intra-articular pathology is adequately addressed.

Once the tear has been assessed arthroscopically, the treatment decision comes to 4 main options: meniscal repair; meniscal debridement/partial meniscectomy; meniscal excision/total meniscectomy; and meniscal replacement.[4] The vast majority of the time surgical decision-making is focused on performing meniscal repair or partial meniscectomy, with the last 2 options reserved for extreme cases. It is important to note that the surgical decision-making process is significantly different for the pediatric and adolescent patient than for the adult: because of the well-documented deleterious effects of meniscectomy on long-term knee function and the increased vascularity of the young person's knee with its attendant enhanced healing potential, preservation of meniscal tissue is of paramount importance in the pediatric patient. Every effort should therefore be made to repair meniscal tears occurring in the red-red and red-white zones in the preadolescent and adolescent knee.

That said, multiple factors related to both the tear and the patient must be considered, including patient age; activity level; surgical history (ie, previous meniscal repair); concomitant injuries; duration of symptoms (tear acuity); the type, size, and location of the tear; and the quality of the meniscal tissue. The "ideal candidate" for surgical repair would be a young patient without history of previous surgery, with an

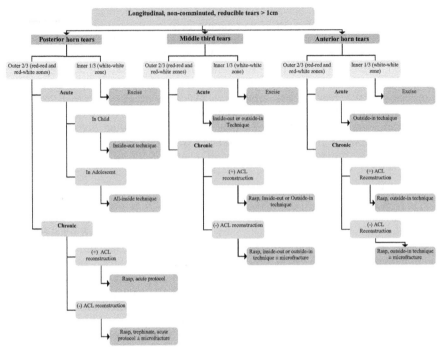

Fig. 1. Treatment algorithm for simple meniscal tears greater than 1 cm in child and adolescent patients.

acute knee injury resulting in a simple, longitudinal meniscal tear, 15 mm in size, occurring in the red-red peripheral zone and associated with an ACL injury.[4] However, this combination of factors rarely exists. In fact, one author's estimate of the rate of meniscal repair performed for isolated meniscal tears occurring in patients younger than 18 years was only 17% (with 83% undergoing partial meniscectomy).[25] Indications for partial meniscectomy include tears confined to the white-white zone (>5 mm from the meniscosynovial junction), tears associated with macerated or degenerative meniscal tissue, irreducible tears, and complex tears with meniscal fragmentation or secondary tearing. An example of an algorithm for treating meniscal injuries in children and adolescents is given in **Fig. 1**.

Once a tear is deemed irreparable, a partial meniscectomy should be performed.[26,27] This can generally be accomplished using a combination of arthroscopic punches to resect torn, unstable tissue. A small arthroscopic shaver may then be used to debride and contour the remaining meniscus. Once this is complete, the meniscus should be probed again to ensure stability of the residual tissue. The primary goal of partial meniscectomy is to maximize meniscal preservation while minimizing the chance of re-tear. Postoperative rehabilitation for patients undergoing partial meniscectomy generally consists of weight-bearing as tolerated, with crutches as needed for assistance for the first several days after surgery. No limits are placed on knee motion, and physical therapy can begin with an immediate focus on regaining motion and strength. Once the operative knee has regained roughly 80% of the strength of the unaffected knee, the patient may be gradually transitioned back into sport.

As stated previously, meniscal tears occurring in the red-red zone or the red-white zone are candidates for meniscal repair. Displaced bucket handle tears should be reduced and evaluated for tissue quality and rim width; bucket handle tears with good quality tissue that are able to be reduced anatomically with a peripheral rim less than 5 mm in width should also undergo repair. Techniques for meniscal repair in the young patient are similar to those performed in adults. The first step is meticulous preparation of the meniscus by debridement of any loose or frayed edges using an arthroscopic shaver. This is followed by rasping of the perimeniscal synovium to stimulate a vascular response and enhance meniscal healing.[28] The next step is then meniscal reduction, ensuring that an anatomic meniscal alignment is achieved prior to suture fixation.

Following meniscal preparation and reduction, repair may then be accomplished using 1 of 4 arthroscopic techniques: all-inside, inside-out, outside-in, and hybrid (a combination). All-inside meniscal repair is performed using 1 of a variety of commercially available fixation devices, such as the FasT-Fix (Smith & Nephew, Andover, MA, USA), the Meniscal Cinch (Arthrex, Naples, FL, USA), and the RapidLoc (Mitek, Westwood, MA, USA). These late-generation implants are suture-based, flexible, and low-profile, a design that minimizes risk of chondral injury while allowing for compression across the meniscal tear. The all-inside devices are well-suited to fixation of longitudinal tears in the red-red or red-white regions of the posterior horn of the meniscus in larger adolescent patients and may obviate the need for the large posterior incisions often required for inside-out repair (**Fig. 2**). However, these devices are not a panacea: because of the possibility of overpenetration of the posterior capsule in a small patient's knee with resultant neurovascular injury, we do not typically use the all-inside technique in younger children. Additionally, there is some concern that the all-inside devices do not provide adequate strength and compression to achieve full meniscal healing.[29] As a result, tears that are unstable may not be good candidates for exclusively all-inside repairs. Hybrid techniques utilizing a combination of all-inside and inside-out suture repairs are commonly employed in this setting.

The inside-out technique uses a double-armed 2-0 polydioxanone suture (PDS) linked by long, flexible needles. In order to effect a meniscal repair, these sutures are passed, in turn, through zone-specific curved cannulas in a vertical mattress fashion. Noyes and Barber-Westin popularized the best-known technique for inside-out meniscal repair in 2002.[30] Using this technique, a series of vertical mattress sutures are placed across the tear, alternating between the inferior and superior surface of the meniscus. Specifically, the first suture pass is 1 to 2 mm peripheral and superior to the tear; the second arm of the same suture is then passed through the meniscus and across the tear itself. A second double-armed suture is then placed 4 to 5 mm from the first, either anteriorly or posteriorly. The first arm of this suture is placed peripheral and inferior to the tear, with the second arm again passing through the meniscus and across the tear. A series of vertical mattress sutures is placed in this alternating fashion until the repair is complete. For repairs performed in the body of the meniscus, a small incision is made in the skin over the suture exit points and blunt dissection is performed down to the level of the joint capsule. An arthroscopic probe is used to harvest the sutures through this incision, and they are then tied down over the joint capsule.

For inside-out repairs performed in the posterior horn of the meniscus, there is a risk of damage to the adjacent neurovascular structures. In these cases, a formal posteromedial or posterolateral approach to the knee with placement of a protective "deflecting" retractor should be made prior to passage of the suture needles. Despite the risk of neurovascular injury with the inside-out technique, it remains the gold standard for meniscal repair as a result of its wide applicability—virtually all areas

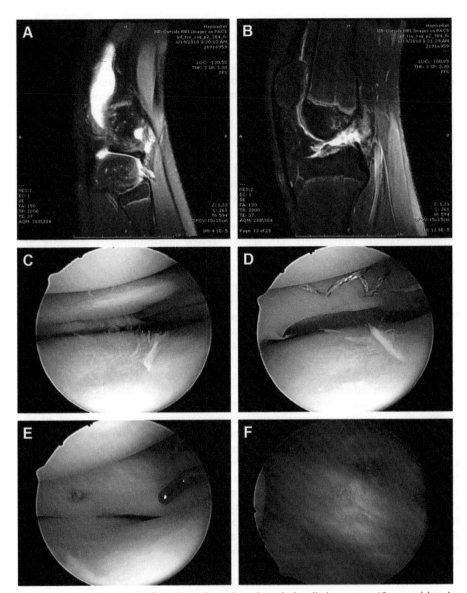

Fig. 2. A longitudinal tear of the lateral meniscus in a skeletally immature 12 year-old male with concomitant ACL tear. *(A)* T2 sagittal MRI demonstrating a tear in the posterior horn of the lateral meniscus. *(B)* T2 sagittal MRI depicting complete concomitant ACL rupture. *(C)* The longitudinal tear in the red-white zone of the posterior horn of the lateral meniscus. *(D)* Placement of a horizontal mattress suture using an all-inside technique. *(E)* The completed repair. *(F)* The final ACL reconstruction performed using a physeal-sparing technique.

of the meniscus can be addressed using this approach—as well as its reliable outcomes.

The outside-in approach is usually reserved for tears located in the anterior horn of the meniscus. Using this technique, two 18-gauge spinal needles are passed percutaneously through the periphery of the intact meniscus and across the tear site into the inner meniscal fragment and then into the central compartment of the knee. A 2-0 PDS suture is then threaded through each needle, and the 2 free suture ends are grasped simultaneously and pulled out the anterior portal. These sutures are tied together outside the knee (a "mulberry knot") and then shuttled back into the joint. Once inside, the knot is pulled taut against the meniscus, holding it in a reduced position. A small skin incision is then made over the suture exit sites and blunt dissection is performed down to the level of the joint capsule. While the meniscal reduction is visualized arthroscopically, the 2 suture ends are tied together over the anterior capsule.

As its name implies, the hybrid technique for meniscal repair employs a combination of the aforementioned techniques. As described, a common scenario for hybrid meniscal repair is the displaced bucket handle tear in an adolescent. In this case, an all-inside device may be used in the posterior horn to minimize the risk of neurovascular injury and avoid the need for a large incision, while the mid-body of the meniscus can be repaired using a traditional inside-out technique.

Repair Augmentation.

If there is concern over the vascularity of the repair—isolated meniscus tears, subacute or chronic tears, tears in the red-white zone—several options to enhance vascularity exist. One such option is trephination, by which an 18- or 22-gauge spinal needle is placed into the meniscus across the tear site and advanced until the peripheral capsule is punctured. This is performed multiple times. The goal of trephination is to create vascular access channels, which connect the meniscal tear with its peripheral blood supply and thereby promote meniscal healing. There is some evidence demonstrating an enhanced healing potential when meniscal repairs are augmented with trephination.[31] Another possible option for maximizing vascular supply to the healing meniscus is the placement of an exogenous fibrin clot.[28,32] Using this technique, approximately 30 mL of blood is obtained from the anesthetized patient from a sterile venipuncture. The blood is placed into a glass container, where it is allowed to clot over a span of roughly 20 minutes while the meniscal repair is performed. Once the repair is complete, the clot is injected directly into the tear site using a large-bore needle and syringe. The efficacy of this technique has also been reported in the literature, and it may be safely used to augment meniscal repair in the young patient.[28,32] Finally, some surgeons have recently advocated the use of microfracture of the femoral notch as a method for improving local vascularity in the setting of meniscal repair.[33]

Postoperative Care

Initial postoperative care for meniscal repairs consists of protected knee mobilization. Both weight-bearing and range of motion (ROM) are restricted in an effort to minimize compressive and shear forces across the repair site. Partial weight-bearing using crutches and a hinged knee brace is the normal postoperative regimen, although the duration of immobilization and the degree to which motion is restricted depend on the type of meniscal tear and the robustness of the repair. Under the supervision of a physical therapist, patients steadily regain knee motion, strength, and endurance. Gradual resumption of impact activity, lateral movement, and sport-specific training follows. Ultimately, patients may return to unrestricted sporting activities once they are entirely asymptomatic and have regained full knee motion and at least 80% of quadriceps strength, usually at 3 to 4 months following surgery.

Possible complications associated with arthroscopy-assisted meniscal repair include infection, arthrofibrosis, deep venous thrombosis, and neurovascular injuries such as peroneal nerve palsy, saphenous neuritis, and complex regional pain syndrome. Chondral injury from protruding implants has also been reported. Perhaps the biggest risk is for failure of the repair, with recurrence of symptoms and the need for secondary surgical procedures.

Outcomes

Outcomes for arthroscopic repair of meniscal tears in the pediatric and adolescent population are highly variable, with success rates ranging from as low as 58% to 100%. In one of the earlier studies to focus on meniscal repair outcomes in the pediatric population, Mintzer and coworkers reported on their clinical results for this procedure. These authors performed 29 meniscal repairs in 26 patients who had an average age of 15.3 years at the time of injury. More than half of this patient population had concomitant ACL tears that were surgically addressed. At an average of 5-year follow-up, there were no instances of clinical failure (a 100% success rate). The average Lysholm score at follow-up was 90 points.[34]

In 1999, Johnson and colleagues reported a 76% clinical success rate at greater than 10-year follow-up for 36 patients undergoing isolated arthroscopy-assisted meniscal repair. These patients had an average age at the time of injury of 20.2 years, and interestingly, had a mean time to surgery of longer than 1 year.[35] Noyes and Barber-Westin reported similar results several years later, when they reviewed the clinical outcomes in 71 knees that had undergone isolated meniscal repairs for tears extending into the central avascular zone. Their study population was composed entirely of patients younger than 20 years. At an average of 51-month follow-up, these authors demonstrated a 75% clinical success rate. This success rate was even higher (87%) when patients who had undergone concomitant ACL reconstruction were considered independently.[30]

More recent authors have been less optimistic about the clinical outcomes for meniscal repair in children and adolescents. In 2007, Accadbled and coworkers reported their results for 12 patients with a mean age of 13 years at the time of injury. At an average of 3-year follow-up, only 58% of patients were completely asymptomatic and fully 25% had undergone reoperation for failure of the primary meniscal repair. Despite this, the average Lysholm score in this group was greater than 96 points.[36] Similarly, Krych and his colleagues reported a clinical success rate of 62% for adolescents undergoing isolated meniscal repair. Their study population consisted of 45 knees in patients with a mean age of 15.8 years followed for an average of 5.8 years postoperatively. These authors noted that while the overall clinical success rate was 62%, it was significantly higher for patients who had simple meniscal tears (80%) and significantly lower for patients with complex tears (13%). Displaced bucket-handle tears had a middling success rate of 68%. These authors identified the rim width and tear complexity as the most important prognostic factors for tear healing.[25]

Most recently, Noyes and colleagues revisited their earlier study and culled a subgroup of patients from the original cohort of 71 knees. Specifically, they identified 31 patients who had undergone 33 meniscal repairs for single, longitudinal meniscal tears with a rim width greater than 4 mm extending into the red-white zone. The mean age of these patients at the time of surgery was 16.4 years, and the average follow-up was 16.8 years. More than half of this patient group had undergone concomitant ACL reconstruction. Using stringent criteria to define clinical success, these authors reported a long-term success rate for meniscal repair of 62%.[37]

Meniscal Tears and ACL Injury

While meniscal tears do occur in isolation in the pediatric and adolescent population, they frequently occur in the setting of ACL injury. Interestingly, there is good evidence to suggest that, just as in the adult population, young patients who undergo meniscal repair at the time of ACL reconstruction enjoy a significantly higher healing rate than those undergoing only meniscal repairs.[38–40] In their study of 51 military cadets who underwent second-look arthroscopy following meniscal repair, Tenuta and Arciero reported a healing rate of 90% for those patients who had undergone a combined ACL reconstruction-meniscal repair versus 57% in those undergoing meniscal repair alone. The average rate of meniscal healing for the entire study population was 81%. Rim width was the most important prognostic factor for meniscal healing, with 3.0 mm set as the cut-off for reliable healing of meniscal tissue. When these authors looked specifically at combined ACL-meniscus repair procedures, they also noted that younger age and decreased time to surgery were significant factors in predicting meniscal healing.[40]

Krych and colleagues reported similar results in their study of clinical outcomes for patients younger than 18 years undergoing concomitant ACL reconstruction and meniscal repair. These authors noted a clinical success rate of 74% at an average of 8 years after surgery. Bucket-handle and complex meniscal tears were routinely associated with poorer clinical outcomes (success rates of 59% and 57%, respectively), while the success rate increased to 84% for simple meniscal tears considered independently.[51] When these authors examined the healing rates of various meniscus tears repaired in conjunction with ACL reconstruction, they found that complex meniscal tears did significantly better in the setting of ACL reconstruction in this younger adolescent and preadolescent population.[39]

DISCOID MENISCUS
Background

The discoid meniscus is a well-described anatomic variant of the lateral meniscus, with an estimated prevalence ranging from less than 1% to upward of 20%.[41–46] There does not seem to be a predilection for gender, although multiple studies have demonstrated racial disparities in the incidence of discoid meniscus, with Asian populations having the highest reported rates. Multiple authors have reported an incidence in the American population ranging from 3% to 6%.[41–46] Unlike a morphologically normal lateral meniscus, the discoid meniscus has both an increased width and an increased thickness, and may be described as "block-like." The discoid meniscus may also have irregular peripheral ligamentous connections that compromise its stability. Importantly, this type of instability is likely more common than previously thought: in 2004, Klingele and his colleagues reported the presence of peripheral rim instability in 28.1% of patients undergoing arthroscopic treatment for discoid meniscus.[47] Good and coworkers subsequently described an even higher rate of meniscal instability associated with the discoid lateral meniscus (77%), highlighting the importance of recognizing and treating this common variant.[43] This finding has subsequently been replicated by other investigators.[48]

Interestingly, there is some recent evidence to suggest that it is not simply the gross morphology of the discoid meniscus that is anomalous, but that its histomorphology is abnormal, too. Building on the work of Atay and colleagues, Papadopoulos and his colleagues recently demonstrated significant disorganization of the circumferential collagen network in the discoid meniscus with an associated heterogeneity in the course of the collagen fibers. They postulated that

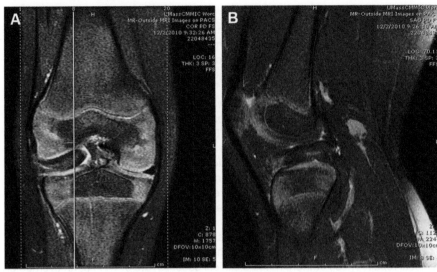

Fig. 3. T2 coronal *(A)* and sagittal *(B)* MRI of a 2+7 year old female with symptomatic discoid meniscus. Note the thickened "block-like" appearance of the lateral meniscus.

this disorganization weakens the collagen ultrastructure of the discoid meniscus, predisposing it to tear.[49,50]

Patients with a discoid meniscus have highly variable presentations. Younger children may present with a painless knee "clunk" and lack of terminal knee extension. "Snapping knee syndrome" is a synonym for an unstable discoid meniscus and is associated with a palpable, audible, or visible "snap" in the knee as it is ranged passively from flexion to extension. Older children, by contrast, more typically present with pain and physical examination findings consistent with a torn meniscus; these include effusion, limited knee motion, lateral joint line tenderness, positive provocative maneuvers such as McMurray and Apley tests, and pain with deep knee flexion.

Plain radiographs of the knee with a discoid meniscus are often normal, although subtle findings such as a widened lateral joint line, squaring of the lateral femoral condyle, and cupping of the lateral tibial plateau may be present. Calcification of the lateral meniscus, hypoplasia of the tibial eminence, and elevation of the fibular head have also been described.[51] MRI is often used as an adjunct to plain radiographs for making the diagnosis of discoid meniscus **(Fig. 3)**. The classic method for MRI diagnosis is to visualize continuity between the posterior and anterior horns of the lateral meniscus (loss of the normal "bow-tie") on 3 consecutive 5-mm sagittal MRI cuts. In addition to diagnosing discoid lateral meniscus, MRI is also useful for identifying concomitant meniscus tears. In one recent study on the role of MRI in diagnosing pediatric knee disorders, MRI was found to have a specificity of 100%, a positive predictive value of 100%, and a negative predictive value of 99.4% when used to diagnose discoid lateral meniscus.[24] However, its sensitivity was only 38.9%, highlighting the importance of a thorough history and physical examination in securing the diagnosis.[24]

Multiple classification systems have been proposed for the discoid meniscus, but the one most widely used is that of Watanabe and colleagues, who described 3 subtypes: (1) type I—complete (disk-shaped) and stable; (2) type II—partial (covers less than 80% of the lateral tibial plateau) and stable; and (3) type III—the "Wrisberg variant," which lacks normal peripheral ligamentous connections and is inherently unstable.[52] Klingele and coworkers recently advocated the use of a simplified classification scheme for discoid menisci based on 3 primary factors: whether the discoid is complete or incomplete; stable or unstable peripherally; and torn or intact.[47,51] This classification scheme seems particularly helpful when devising a surgical treatment strategy.

Historically, the preferred treatment for symptomatic discoid menisci was total or subtotal meniscectomy. In recent years, however, the evidence against performing this type of procedure in children and young adults has continued to mount, with the majority of mid- and long-term outcomes studies demonstrating early degenerative changes radiographically following these procedures.[11–14,17–19,53,54] Osteochondritis dissecans lesions of the lateral femoral condyle following excision of a discoid meniscus have also been reported.[55] While surgical salvage techniques such as meniscal allograft transplantation do exist, they tend to be more technically demanding with incompletely understood outcomes.[56,57] As a result, methods for treating the discoid meniscus have shifted away from the surgically aggressive to the more conservative current standard of care. Today, the primary goal of surgical intervention is to maximize knee stability and function by restoring anatomic dimensions to the lateral meniscus and repairing torn or unstable residual meniscal tissue. Meniscal saucerization with stabilization and repair as deemed necessary intraoperatively has effectively supplanted meniscectomy in the treatment of the discoid meniscus.[58,59]

Treatment

Nonsurgical management of the discoid meniscus is reserved for those that are asymptomatic or incidentally found. For knees that are symptomatic, surgical treatment is indicated. This consists first of a diagnostic knee arthroscopy of the affected knee to identify concomitant intra-articular pathology; to determine the type of discoid meniscus (complete or incomplete); to assess the overall stability of the meniscus; and to note the presence of an associated meniscal tear (**Fig. 4**A).

Arthroscopic meniscal saucerization is then performed (see **Fig. 4B–C**). This is often begun with the knee in flexion, because it may be difficult to gain access to the lateral compartment as a result of the thickened, abnormal meniscal tissue. Saucerization begins centrally in the meniscus and may be performed using a combination of arthroscopic punches and a small motorized shaver. Once the central area of meniscal tissue is removed, the knee may be placed into the standard figure-of-four position to complete the saucerization. In some cases, a meniscal knife may be used to assist in resection and contouring of the abnormal tissue. Saucerization of the discoid tissue is performed until a peripheral rim of roughly 6 to 8 mm remains. This residual tissue width may be estimated using the arthroscopic probe, whose typical length from the curve to the tip is 7 mm. Another method of assessing the appropriate amount of meniscal resection is to examine the lateral femoral condyle for an indentation that indicates an area of chronic abnormal contact between the overlarge meniscus and the adjacent condyle. Meniscal resection may be performed to this line of demarcation.

Once the discoid meniscal saucerization is complete, the remaining meniscal tissue should be assessed for evidence of instability or tearing (see **Fig. 4D**). Instability may be defined as more than 11 mm of meniscal excursion; the ability to translate the anterior meniscal horn fully onto the posterior tibial plateau; or the ability to fully avert the lateral meniscus.[60] Similarly, the meniscus should be evaluated for the presence and type of meniscal tears. Meniscal instability, if present, should be addressed with surgical stabilization of the meniscus to the capsule. Typically, an inside-out repair

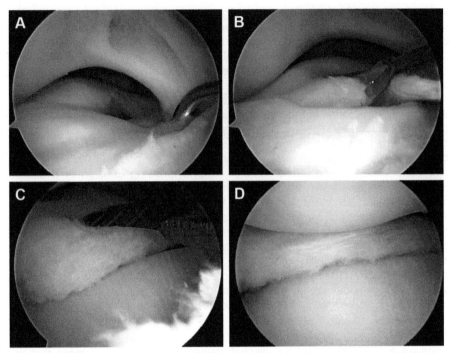

Fig. 4. Arthroscopic saucerization of a complete, stable discoid lateral meniscus. *(A)* Appearance of the discoid meniscus prior to resection. *(B)* An arthroscopic punch is used to initiate resection of the abnormal tissue. *(C)* A meniscal knife may be used for meniscal resection and contouring. *(D)* The final appearance of the lateral meniscus following arthroscopic saucerization. Note that the residual tissue should be meticulously probed to ensure that it is stable peripherally.

using zone-specific cannulas to place multiple sutures across the meniscocapsular junction is performed. In larger knees, an all-inside technique using a commercially available meniscal repair device may also be used. For concomitant meniscal tears that are present in the central avascular zone or consist of poor quality tissue, simple debridement with a small arthroscopic shaver is adequate. However, meniscal tears that extend into the periphery merit formal repair, which may be achieved through one of the aforementioned arthroscopic techniques.

Postoperative Care

Immediate postoperative care is determined at the time of surgery. Patients who undergo arthroscopic meniscal saucerization alone are encouraged to bear weight as tolerated immediately on the affected leg with unrestricted knee range of motion. Patients who require meniscal stabilization and/or meniscal repair with the saucerization procedure are given a hinged knee brace and crutches for protection of knee motion and weight-bearing for a period of 4 to 6 weeks postoperatively. Formal physical therapy is begun within 1 to 2 weeks postoperatively with the goal of gradual improvement in knee strength, motion, and endurance. Once knee strength and motion have been restored, a supervised return to sport is permitted, usually at 3 to 4 months postoperative.

Outcomes

Clinical and functional outcomes for patients who have undergone surgical treatment for discoid meniscus are variable and are likely dependent upon the surgical procedure performed. As previously noted, young patients treated with total meniscectomy are at risk for developing early degenerative changes in the knee.[10,13,15,16,19,20] One example of this causative association was published in 1998 by Räber and colleagues, who reported their results for total meniscectomy performed for symptomatic discoid meniscus in 17 knees. At an average of 19.8-year follow-up, these authors noted that more than 50% of their patients had clinical symptoms of arthritis, with two-thirds of the patients evidencing radiographic changes of osteoarthritis such as flattening of the lateral femoral condyle.[19]

Several authors have reported their results with partial meniscectomy for discoid meniscus. As early as 1989, Vandermeer and Cunningham reported their results with arthroscopic meniscal saucerization performed in 22 patients. At an average of 54-month follow-up, these authors noted a 28% reoperation rate, with only 64% of patients resuming a "normal" activity level postoperatively.[54] Aglietti and coworkers reported on their results of arthroscopic lateral meniscectomy performed for discoid meniscus; at an average follow-up of 10 years postoperatively, these authors noted radiographic changes including lateral compartment osteophyte formation and lateral joint space narrowing at rates of 47% and 65%, respectively.[11] In 2003, Atay et al reported on their results of partial meniscectomy performed in 34 knees. At an average of 5.6 years postoperatively, they found that the vast majority of patients (85%) had excellent or good outcomes. These authors did, however, note a statistically significant difference in the presence of radiographic changes (eg, lateral femoral condyle flattening) in the postmeniscectomy knees.[12] Finally, Og̈üt and colleagues reported their 4.5-year outcomes in 11 knees treated with partial meniscectomy for symptomatic discoid meniscus. These authors found that 100% of patients had good or excellent clinical outcomes, with no patient having degenerative changes on radiographs.[17]

Information on arthroscopic meniscal saucerization performed with concomitant stabilization is available, although there is a paucity of long-term outcomes data for these patients. In their case series of 5 patients with torn discoid lateral menisci treated with partial meniscectomy and suture repair, Adachi and colleagues reported "excellent" outcomes in 4 of 5 patients evaluated 2 years postoperatively with an average improvement in Lysholm score of 12.4 points (83.4 points average preoperative score to 95.8 points average postoperative score).[56] In 2007, Good and coworkers reported on their series of 21 patients who had undergone arthroscopic saucerization with associated meniscal stabilization being performed in more than three-quarters of patients. At an average 37.4-month follow-up, all patients had regained knee flexion beyond 135°, although 3 patients reported persistent knee pain and 4 patients had mechanical symptoms.[43] Finally, in 2008, Ahn and his colleagues reported on their larger series of 77 patients treated in a similar fashion with arthroscopic partial meniscectomy and suture repair. At a mid-term follow-up of 51 months, these authors reported a 100% rate of return to full activities with no incidence of reoperation; their average improvement in Lysholm score was 17 points (78.5 preoperative mean score to 95.5 postoperatively).[59]

MENISCAL INSTABILITY/HYPERMOBILITY
Background

While significantly rarer than traumatic meniscal tears or discoid lateral meniscus, meniscal instability is a well-described phenomenon in the young patient. In fact, there are multiple case reports of patients presenting with a "locked knee" without physical or radiographic evidence of meniscal injury.[61-65] In many of these cases, subsequent MRI or knee arthroscopy has been used to identify the source of dysfunction as meniscal instability, due to either deficiency or tearing of the normal meniscocapsular attachments. Hypermobility of both the lateral meniscus (usually the posterior horn) and medial meniscus (usually the anterior horn) has been described in the literature.[61-65]

Patients with meniscal instability typically present with intermittent mechanical symptoms, including locking of the knee, which often requires some sort of manipulation or reduction maneuver to alleviate the symptoms. Trauma or injury to the knee may be elicited as part of the patient's history, but more often meniscal instability is not associated with any specific injury. Physical examination of the affected knee may reveal findings similar to a meniscal tear—effusion, joint line tenderness, loss of joint motion, and positive provocative maneuvers such as the McMurray's test—but in the absence of a recent locking episode, the appearance of the knee may be quite normal. Similarly, plain radiographs and MRI are unlikely to reveal frank abnormality. The exception to this may be the patient with an acutely disrupted popliteomeniscal fasciculus: one recent report of a series of 3 cases of unstable lateral menisci found that a disruption of the lateral popliteo-meniscal fasciculi was evident on the MRI in all 3 patients, despite an initial MRI reading of "normal" by the referring institution.[65]

Treatment

Patients with symptomatic, recurrent meniscal hypermobility benefit from surgical intervention. In general, this consists of arthroscopic stabilization of the unstable meniscus by suturing it to the adjacent joint capsule. Arthroscopic stabilization techniques may vary somewhat, but inside-out, all-inside, and hybrid constructs repair constructs are all viable surgical options. In one recent case report of a medial meniscal dislocation, open surgical reconstruction of the deficient meniscocapsular ligaments was performed using suture anchors and a capsular reefing technique.[61] Postoperative rehabilitation is similar to that for a standard meniscal repair, consisting of an initial period of protected weight-bearing and relative immobilization followed by a gradual, supervised return to activity. Because meniscal hypermobility occurs only infrequently, clinical outcomes data are limited.

SUMMARY

Meniscal injury is an increasingly recognized phenomenon in children and adolescents. Acute, traumatic tears of the meniscus occur with some frequency in the young athlete and may be associated with concomitant intra-articular pathology, including ACL injury. Anatomic meniscal variants such as the lateral discoid meniscus are predisposed to tearing, which may occur in the absence of significant trauma. Rare meniscal pathology, including hypermobility of the meniscus, has also been reported in the literature. In many cases of meniscal injury in the child and adolescent, a detailed history and physical examination are adequate for making the diagnosis of meniscal tear. However, because children are often less able to accurately verbalize their symptoms and cooperate with examinations, adjunctive diagnostic imaging such as MRI may be extremely helpful in securing the diagnosis.

Because the meniscus in children and adolescents is more vascular than the adult meniscus, it has been widely postulated that the potential for meniscal healing in the young person is enhanced. Additionally, numerous studies have demonstrated the deleterious effects of meniscectomy on long-term knee function. As a result, meniscal tears in the preadolescent and adolescent age groups are frequently treated with arthroscopic-assisted meniscal repair using a variety of surgical approaches including outside-in, inside-out, all-inside, and hybrid techniques. Occasionally, these repairs may be augmented by meniscal trephination, microfracture of the femoral notch, and fibrin clot application to maximize healing potential. Symptomatic lateral discoid menisci are treated with arthroscopic saucerization with meniscal repair and/or stabilization performed as deemed necessary intraoperatively. Hypermobility or instability of the meniscus is rare, but when it does occur and is symptomatic, it should be treated with arthroscopic meniscal stabilization.

Certain factors optimize the ability of meniscal tears to heal and these include: younger age; acuity of injury; concomitant ACL injury; simple tear type; smaller tear size; and peripheral location of tear (decreased rim width). Some types of meniscal tears are simply not amenable to surgical repair and, in these instances, judicious partial meniscectomy is indicated. Algorithms exist to help guide surgical decision-making, although definitive treatment for meniscal tears in the young patient should always be individualized, taking into account the patient's age, surgical history, concomitant injuries, and activity level.

REFERENCES

1. Conn JM, Annest JL, Gilchrist J. Sports and recreation related injury episodes in the US population, 1997-99. Inj Prev 2003;9:117–23.
2. Stanitski CL, Harvell JC, Fu F. Observations on acute knee hemarthrosis in children and adolescents. J Pediatr Orthop 1993;13:506–10.
3. Vaquero J, Vidal C, Cubillo A. Intra-articular traumatic disorders of the knee in children and adolescents. Clin Orthop Relat Res 2005;432:97–106.
4. Brown TD, Davis JT. Meniscal injury in the skeletally immature patient. In: Micheli LJ, Kocher MS, editors. The Pediatric and Adolescent Knee. Philadelphia: Elsevier; 2006. p. 236–59.
5. Clark CR, Ogden JA. Development of the menisci of the human knee joint. Morphological changes and their potential role in childhood meniscal injury. J Bone Joint Surg Am 1983;65:538–47.
6. Fithian DC, Kelly MA, Mow VC. Material properties and structure-function relationships in the menisci. Clin Orthop Relat Res 1990;252:19–31.
7. McDevitt CA, Webber RJ. The ultrastructure and biochemistry of meniscal cartilage. Clin Orthop Relat Res 1990;252:8–18.
8. Ahmed AM, Burke DL. In-vitro measurement of static pressure distribution in synovial joints—Part I: tibial surface of the knee. J Biomech Eng 1983;105:216–25.
9. Baratz ME, Fu FH, Mengato R. Meniscal tears: the effect of meniscectomy and of repair on intra-articular contact areas and stress in the human knee. A preliminary report. Am J Sports Med 1986;14:270–5.
10. Abdon P, Turner MS, Pettersson H, et al. A long-term follow-up study of total meniscectomy in children. Clin Orthop Relat Res 1990;257:166–70.
11. Aglietti P, Bertini FA, Buzzi R, et al. Arthroscopic meniscectomy for discoid lateral meniscus in children and adolescents: 10-year follow-up. Am J Knee Surg 1999;12: 83–7.
12. Atay OA, Doral MN, Leblebicioglu G, et al. Management of discoid lateral meniscus tears: observations in 34 knees. Arthroscopy 2003;19:346–52.
13. Habata T, Uematsu K, Kasanami R, et al. Long-term clinical and radiographic follow-up of total resection for discoid lateral meniscus. Arthroscopy 2006;22(12): 1339–43.

14. Lee DH, Kim TH, Kim JM, et al. Results of subtotal/total or partial meniscectomy for discoid lateral meniscus in children. Arthroscopy 2009;25:496–503.
15. Manzione M, Pizzutillo PD, Peoples AB, et al. Meniscectomy in children: a long-term follow-up study. Am J Sports Med 1983;11:111–5.
16. Medlar RC, Mandiberg JJ, Lyne ED. Meniscectomies in children. Report of long-term results (mean, 8.3 years) of 26 children. Am J Sports Med 1980;8:87–92.
17. Ogut T, Kesmezacar H, Akgun I, et al. Arthroscopic meniscectomy for discoid lateral meniscus in children and adolescents: 4.5 year follow-up. J Pediatr Orthop B 2003;12:390–7.
18. Okazaki K, Miura H, Matsuda S, et al. Arthroscopic resection of the discoid lateral meniscus: long-term follow-up for 16 years. Arthroscopy 2006;22:967–71.
19. Raber DA, Friederich NF, Hefti F. Discoid lateral meniscus in children. Long-term follow-up after total meniscectomy. J Bone Joint Surg Am 1998;80:1579–86.
20. Wroble RR, Henderson RC, Campion ER, et al. Meniscectomy in children and adolescents. A long-term follow-up study. Clin Orthop Relat Res 1992;279:180–9.
21. Arnoczky SP, Warren RF. The microvasculature of the meniscus and its response to injury. An experimental study in the dog. Am J Sports Med 1983;11:131–41.
22. King D. The healing of semilunar cartilages 1936. Clin Orthop Relat Res 1990;252: 4–7.
23. Bloome DM, Blevins FT, Paletta GA Jr, et al. Meniscal repair in very young children. Arthroscopy 2000;16:545–9.
24. Kocher MS, DiCanzio J, Zurakowski D, et al. Diagnostic performance of clinical examination and selective magnetic resonance imaging in the evaluation of intra-articular knee disorders in children and adolescents. Am J Sports Med 2001;29: 292–6.
25. Krych AJ, McIntosh AL, Voll AE, et al. Arthroscopic repair of isolated meniscal tears in patients 18 years and younger. Am J Sports Med 2008;36:1283–9.
26. DeHaven KE. Meniscus repair. Am J Sports Med 1999;27:242–50.
27. Sgaglione NA, Steadman JR, Shaffer B, et al. Current concepts in meniscus surgery: resection to replacement. Arthroscopy 2003;19(Suppl 1):161–88.
28. Henning CE, Lynch MA, Clark JR. Vascularity for healing of meniscus repairs. Arthroscopy 1987;3:13–8.
29. Hospodar SJ, Schmitz MR, Golish SR, et al. FasT-Fix versus inside-out suture meniscal repair in the goat model. Am J Sports Med 2009;37:330–3.
30. Noyes FR, Barber-Westin SD. Arthroscopic repair of meniscal tears extending into the avascular zone in patients younger than twenty years of age. Am J Sports Med 2002;30:589–600.
31. Zhang Z, Arnold JA, Williams T, et al. Repairs by trephination and suturing of longitudinal injuries in the avascular area of the meniscus in goats. Am J Sports Med 1995;23:35–41.
32. Arnoczky SP, Warren RF, Spivak JM. Meniscal repair using an exogenous fibrin clot. An experimental study in dogs. J Bone Joint Surg Am 1988;70:1209–17.
33. Freedman KB, Nho SJ, Cole BJ. Marrow stimulating technique to augment meniscus repair. Arthroscopy 2003;19:794–8.
34. Mintzer CM, Richmond JC, Taylor J. Meniscal repair in the young athlete. Am J Sports Med 1998;26:630–3.
35. Johnson MJ, Lucas GL, Dusek JK, et al. Isolated arthroscopic meniscal repair: a long-term outcome study (more than 10 years). Am J Sports Med 1999;27:44–9.
36. Accadbled F, Cassard X, Sales de Gauzy J, et al. Meniscal tears in children and adolescents: results of operative treatment. J Pediatr Orthop B 2007;16:56–60.

37. Noyes FR, Chen RC, Barber-Westin SD, et al. Greater than 10-year results of red-white longitudinal meniscus repairs in patients 20 years of age or younger. Am J Sports Med 2011;39(5):1008–17.

38. Asahina S, Muneta T, Yamamoto H. Arthroscopic meniscal repair in conjunction with anterior cruciate ligament reconstruction: factors affecting the healing rate. Arthroscopy 1996;12:541–5.

39. Krych AJ, Pitts RT, Dajani KA, et al. Surgical repair of meniscal tears with concomitant anterior cruciate ligament reconstruction in patients 18 years and younger. Am J Sports Med 2010;38:976–82.

40. Tenuta JJ, Arciero RA. Arthroscopic evaluation of meniscal repairs. Factors that effect healing. Am J Sports Med 1994;22:797–802.

41. Bellier G, Dupont JY, Larrain M, et al. Lateral discoid menisci in children. Arthroscopy 1989;5:52–6.

42. Dickhaut SC, DeLee JC. The discoid lateral-meniscus syndrome. J Bone Joint Surg Am 1982;64:1068–73.

43. Good CR, Green DW, Griffith MH, et al. Arthroscopic treatment of symptomatic discoid meniscus in children: classification, technique, and results. Arthroscopy 2007;23:157–63.

44. Ikeuchi H. Arthroscopic treatment of the discoid lateral meniscus. Technique and long-term results. Clin Orthop Relat Res 1982;167:19–28.

45. Kramer DE, Micheli LJ. Meniscal tears and discoid meniscus in children: diagnosis and treatment. J Am Acad Orthop Surg 2009;17:698–707.

46. Rao PS, Rao SK, Paul R. Clinical, radiologic, and arthroscopic assessment of discoid lateral meniscus. Arthroscopy 2001;17:275–7.

47. Klingele KE, Kocher MS, Hresko MT, et al. Discoid lateral meniscus: prevalence of peripheral rim instability. J Pediatr Orthop 2004;24:79–82.

48. Yoo WJ, Choi IH, Chung CY, et al. Discoid lateral meniscus in children: limited knee extension and meniscal instability in the posterior segment. J Pediatr Orthop 2008; 28:544–8.

49. Atay OA, Pekmezci M, Doral MN, et al. Discoid meniscus: an ultrastructural study with transmission electron microscopy. Am J Sports Med 2007;35:475–8.

50. Papadopoulos A, Kirkos JM, Kapetanos GA. Histomorphologic study of discoid meniscus. Arthroscopy 2009;25:262–8.

51. Kocher MS, Klingele K, Rassman SO. Meniscal disorders: normal, discoid, and cysts. Orthop Clin North Am 2003;34:329–40.

52. Watanabe M, Takeda S, Ikeuchi H. Atlas of Arthroscopy. 3rd edition. Tokyo (Japan): Igaku-Shoin; 1979.

53. Aichroth PM, Patel DV, Marx CL. Congenital discoid lateral meniscus in children. A follow-up study and evolution of management. J Bone Joint Surg Br 1991;73:932–6.

54. Vandermeer RD, Cunningham FK. Arthroscopic treatment of the discoid lateral meniscus: results of long-term follow-up. Arthroscopy 1989;5:101–9.

55. Mizuta H, Nakamura E, Otsuka Y, et al. Osteochondritis dissecans of the lateral femoral condyle following total resection of the discoid lateral meniscus. Arthroscopy 2001;17:608–12.

56. Cole BJ, Dennis MG, Lee SJ, et al. Prospective evaluation of allograft meniscus transplantation: a minimum 2-year follow-up. Am J Sports Med 2006;34:919–27.

57. Kim JM, Bin SI. Meniscal allograft transplantation after total meniscectomy of torn discoid lateral meniscus. Arthroscopy 2006;22(12):1344–50,e1.

58. Adachi N, Ochi M, Uchio Y, et al. Torn discoid lateral meniscus treated using partial central meniscectomy and suture of the peripheral tear. Arthroscopy 2004;20:536–42.

59. Ahn JH, Lee SH, Yoo JC, et al. Arthroscopic partial meniscectomy with repair of the peripheral tear for symptomatic discoid lateral meniscus in children: results of minimum 2 years of follow-up. Arthroscopy 2008;24:888–98.
60. Weiss JM. Discoid Lateral Meniscus Saucerization and Stabilization. In: Tolo VT, Skaggs DL, editors. Masters Techniques in Pediatric Orthopaedic Surgery. Philadelphia: Lippincott Williams & Wilkins; 2008. p. 289–96.
61. Chan SK, Robb CA, Singh T, et al. Medial dislocation of the medial meniscus. J Bone Joint Surg Br 2010;92:155–7.
62. Garofalo R, Kombot C, Borens O, et al. Locking knee caused by subluxation of the posterior horn of the lateral meniscus. Knee Surg Sports Traumatol Arthrosc 2005; 13:569–71.
63. George M, Wall EJ. Locked knee caused by meniscal subluxation: magnetic resonance imaging and arthroscopic verification. Arthroscopy 2003;19:885–8.
64. Lyle NJ, Sampson MA, Barrett DS. MRI of intermittent meniscal dislocation in the knee. Br J Radiol 2009;82:374–9.
65. Simonian PT, Sussmann PS, Wickiewicz TL, et al. Popliteomeniscal fasciculi and the unstable lateral meniscus: clinical correlation and magnetic resonance diagnosis. Arthroscopy 1997;13:590–6.

Return to Sport After Meniscal Repair

Anthony M. Barcia, MD[a],*, Erick J. Kozlowski, BS, ATC[b],
John M. Tokish, MD[a]

KEYWORDS

- Meniscus • Meniscal repair • Rehabilitation • Therapy
- Return to sport

Preservation of meniscal function is among the most important goals in knee surgery. Loss of this function after meniscal injury and treatment with meniscectomy has long been recognized to play a major role in the deterioration in knee function and the development of degenerative joint disease.[1,2] Therefore, surgeons have become more aggressive with meniscal repair and adjunctive procedures to promote healing in meniscal surgery.[3]

Compared to the rehabilitation period after meniscectomy, the period of restricted motion and limitation of knee function after meniscal repair is longer and more complex. The repair must be protected, and there are certainly activities that are avoided during the healing process in order to optimize healing. But it is equally critical that the repair not be neglected—immobilization and disuse have a cost, and a postoperative knee that is overprotected may function no better than the preoperative knee with a meniscus tear. Thus, if the ultimate outcome measure is return to sport, then a healed meniscus is only the beginning. It must function within a knee and kinetic chain that has regained muscular control, proprioception, and confidence of use. Much of this chain can continue to be strengthened even during the most protective postoperative phases, so that when healing of the meniscus is achieved, the knee can be placed back into a well-functioning kinetic chain, allowing parallel protection and mobilization to simultaneously take place. It is this broader aspect of rehabilitation that is often misunderstood by the orthopedist and will be the focus of this article.

Traditional postoperative rehabilitation programs are generally divided into phases. The earliest phase after meniscus repair was often governed by specific criteria such as wound healing, resolution of effusion, pain control, range of motion, and evidence

The authors have nothing to disclose.
[a] Tripler Army Medical Center, 1 Jarrett White Road, Honolulu, HI 96859-5000, USA
[b] United States Air Force Academy, 2304 Cadet Drive, Suite 3100, U.S. Air Force Academy, CO 80840-5016, USA
* Corresponding author.
E-mail address: anthony.m.barcia@us.army.mil

of muscular return. The postoperative involvement with the surgeon was governed by these phases, with each visit to the surgeon at the time where the goals of the phase were expected to be met. A typical progression of this phase may have been non–weight bearing and restricted motion for 6 weeks, with the first postoperative visit with the surgeon at 2 weeks to ensure wound healing and compliance with these restrictions. The next visit at around 6 weeks postoperatively would ensure the knee was "ready" to begin therapy which usually meant progression of weight bearing, and restoration of range of motion. Next, the patient would be brought back at around 3 months with a goal for the patient to have achieved full range of motion and be walking normally. If this was accomplished, the surgeon might clear the patient for some sort of strengthening program and stress the importance of quadriceps retraining. One more visit at perhaps 4 to 5 months was typical to ensure good muscle tone and bulk, at which time a patient would be cleared to return to sport.

There are several problems with this traditional approach. First, the patient's progression is based on assumptions that are only checked at 6-week intervals. This approach does not take into account individual patient responses, and "progress" is monitored by the surgeon, who generally does not evaluate other aspects of rehabilitation like core strength and kinetic chain maintenance. Second, the assumptions of the effect of weight bearing and immobilization during the first 6 weeks after surgery may not be correct. Third, there is a cost in terms of muscular rhythm, and dynamic strengthening that may take months to recover from with this approach. Finally, even at the completion of this type of program, when the surgeon has "cleared" the patient for return to sport, there has been no assessment of any dynamic aspect of performance. Because return to sport is a dynamic event, these traditional programs stopped well short of the goal of the operation in the first place.

COMPARING TRADITIONAL AND ACCELERATED PRINCIPLES

There is no widely accepted or validated rehabilitation algorithm for patients who have undergone meniscus repair. The necessity of the more conservative rehabilitation measures has been brought into question by the success of accelerated rehabilitation protocols, which have demonstrated no detriment when more aggressive approaches are employed. While recent data indicate that the accelerated rehabilitation programs are safe and at least as effective as more conservative approaches, the rehabilitation plan should be tailored individually, taking into account the type of tear and concurrent injuries. While we advocate an aggressive program to optimize the kinetic chain during healing, these factors must be heeded to ensure reliable healing. In the protection phase of the program, when the meniscus is not healed, the most controversial factors are immobilization and weight bearing status. While these questions have not been definitively answered, there has been much work done to examine their effects on meniscal healing.

IMMOBILIZATION

Both mechanical and biologic factors are critical in the postoperative decisions regarding immobilization, weight bearing, motion, and activity. Immobilization in full extension after meniscal repair traditionally has been recommended by multiple authors to reapproximate longitudinal tears of the meniscus.[4,5] Animal models have shown that the effect of immobilization has a greater effect on meniscus healing than the use of suture or approach of repair with impressive healing rates using only immobilization.[6,7] However, Dowdy and colleagues showed that immobilization after meniscus repair impaired the biologic healing of repaired meniscus.[8] Furthermore, the benefits of passive motion on the healing of articular cartilage have been well documented in an animal model.[9] Thus, in the setting where meniscal repair is combined with other procedures such as treatment of a chondral defect, one must carefully weigh the cost of immobilization. Finally, significant quadriceps atrophy occurs with immobilization, which may contribute to the delay in the return to sport of the injured athlete.[10]

The traditional recommendation of a period of decreased mobility consisting of 4 to 6 weeks was proposed to protect the healing meniscus. The rationale for conservative rehabilitation was protecting the repair and allowing formation of a fibrovascular scar.[11] More recently, however, the literature has failed to show any deleterious effect of early range of motion after meniscal repair leading many to advocate for accelerated rehabilitation protocol.[12–14] Barber and colleagues reported no differences in healing rates and outcomes in patients who followed a conventional protective rehabilitation compared with patients who were allowed immediate weight bearing, full range of motion without a brace, unlimited exercise, and an early return to pivoting-type sports.[15] While short-term outcome data exist, long-term data are still lacking.

WEIGHT BEARING

Weight bearing in full extension with limited motion may have stimulating effects on the healing response.[16] Additionally, in repaired bucket handle tears, weight bearing actually reduces and stabilizes the meniscus.[17] Conversely, activity that involves tibiofemoral loads across a flexed knee has been shown to cause compressive and shear loads. A 4-fold increase in pressure on the posterior horn of the meniscus was shown when weight bearing in 90° of flexion compared to full extension.[18]

Weight bearing in full extension has not been shown to put a repaired meniscus at risk, except in the relatively unusual cases of a complete radial tear or posterior root tear, where there is a complete transection of the circumferential fibers.[19] Large excursions of the meniscus are seen with tibial rotation and unacceptable levels of compressive stresses are associated with terminal flexion, making both deep squats and tibial rotation concerning for the first 12 weeks after meniscal repair. Accelerated protocols with more aggressive rehabilitation have been proposed and as yet have failed to show a significantly worse affect with this approach, but more data are necessary to clarify which restrictions may be safely lifted without deleterious effect.[20]

ACCELERATED REHABILITATION PROTOCOLS

Mariani and coworkers examined 22 meniscal repair patients, undergoing simultaneous ACL reconstruction, who were allowed to proceed to full weight bearing in extension as soon as tolerated in a locked brace only during ambulation for the first 4 weeks, with no other restrictions in active or passive range of motion.[21] Closed chain kinetic exercises, low resistance stationary cycling, and swimming were started at 2 to 4 weeks postoperatively. At 4 weeks, progressive resistance exercise was initiated, followed by running and cycling at 2 months and unrestricted return to sport without a functional brace at 6 months postoperatively. Patients were evaluated clinically and with MRI at an average of 28 months postoperatively and only 3 of 22 were found to have symptomatic and MRI evidence of failure, leading the authors to propose the safety of this more aggressive approach.

Shelbourne and colleagues prospectively evaluated 65 patients who underwent an isolated meniscal repair for displaced bucket handle tears without a concurrent ACL reconstruction.[2] Initially the authors treated 17 patients with a conservative approach (with restricted range of motion and weight bearing for 6 weeks, allowing return to full activity only after 4 to 6 months of protected activity) but found that during this time some patients progressed more rapidly than others. It was noted that those who progressed more rapidly were not complying with the rehabilitation guidelines and had voluntarily accelerated their activity. As a result of these observations, the authors adopted an accelerated protocol that encouraged early weight bearing and range of motion as tolerated in the immediate postoperative period. The revised protocol also emphasized prevention of intra-articular effusion and swelling and allowed return to full activity when the following were attained: full range of motion, at least 75% strength of the nonoperative leg, and when they had completed a functional running program. Patients in the accelerated group returned to sport faster (10 vs 20 weeks) and had no significant difference in the rate of failure or in functional level as assessed by Lysholm scores, modified Noyes score, or self-evaluation. The authors concluded that most of the activity restrictions imposed by conventional rehabilitation protocols may not be necessary and that an accelerated rehabilitation protocol is safe.

SUPERVISED VERSUS UNSUPERVISED THERAPY

Multiple studies assessing return to sport after partial meniscectomy have compared a well-planned, unsupervised rehabilitation program with supervised physical therapy. Jokl and coworkers found no significant difference between the 2 groups, whereas Moffet and colleagues demonstrated a more rapid recovery of the quadriceps femoris muscle with supervised therapy.[22,23] It has been shown that an interval of 4 to 6 weeks is required for the quadriceps femoris muscle to return to preoperative isokinetic strength after partial meniscectomy and an interval of 4 weeks was required for the hamstrings.[24] It should be noted that return to sport was not assessed as an outcome in these studies, and one would expect that more aggressive demands on the athletic knee, especially after meniscal repair, would benefit to an even greater extent with supervised therapy, but no study exists that evaluates return to sport with unsupervised versus supervised rehabilitation after meniscal repair.

OPTIMIZATION OF RETURN TO SPORT

It is important to understand that optimal return to sport does not necessarily mean the fastest return to sport possible. A college football player who undergoes a meniscal repair in January may be managed differently than one who has the same surgery in May, if the ultimate goal is to return for the following season. This demonstrates the point of knowing not just the pathology treated in the operating room but to whom that pathology belongs and what his or her postoperative goals, resources, and restrictions bring to bear on return to sport. We rely on a close partnership with our physical therapists and athletic trainers. These specialists see the athlete on a daily basis and learn to recognize the patient's kinetic flaws, compensations, and progression far better than the orthopedist.

Our program after meniscal repair actually begins preoperatively. Patients are taught core strengthening techniques such as bridges and planks and are taught to recognize how to "draw in" the abdominal musculature to optimize the core (**Fig. 1**). These exercises are more than abdominal crunches and are carried on throughout the postoperative course, modified but uninterrupted, to ensure maintenance of core strength.

At the completion of the operation, the patient is immobilized in full extension with a brace. This step is less for protection than encouraging full extension, and after the patient is alert we allow for removal to begin range of motion depending on repair

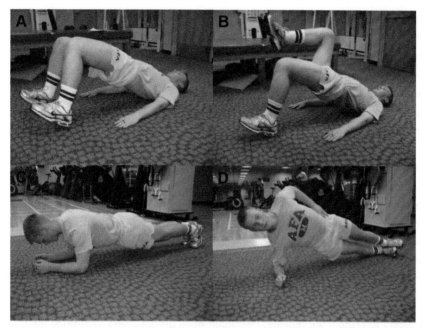

Fig. 1. Core strengthening techniques. These exercises are designed to enhance core stability and promote proper transfer of energy throughout the kinetic chain. This routine begins preoperatively and is continued throughout the postoperative rehabilitation. (*A*) Double leg gluteus bridge, (*B*) single leg gluteus bridge, (*C*) double leg prone bridge, (*D*) side bridge.

type. In certain repairs, such as meniscal root avulsions and radial tears, we limit flexion to 90°, as deep flexion has been shown to increase forces across the meniscus. We allow immediate weight bearing in full extension, except in tear patterns where axial loads will distract the repair, such as in radial and complex tears. Pain control and effusion management are critical steps in the early postoperative phase, and we useregional anesthesia and cooling/compression devices in most cases. Our athletes visit with the athletic trainer on postoperative day 1, where an initial evaluation is done, and core strengthening is resumed. Compression wrapping, passive patellar mobilization, and early quad sets are also instructed and supervised.

CRITERIA FOR INITIATING RETURN TO SPORT

It is important to define in advance the criteria that are used for allowing an athlete to advance from the initial rehabilitation phase to the final stages of return to sport. An athlete who returns to high-level activity before functional stability has been achieved is at an increased risk for a poor outcome.[25] These baseline criteria are summarized in **Box 1** and include the absence of effusion, full range of motion, and good quadriceps control and strength. The operative leg strength should be recovered to at least 70% in terms of extension, flexion, and leg press, compared to the contralateral leg, before resuming sport after meniscal repair. Importantly, the athlete should feel "ready" to progress to the more active and dynamic phase with Single Alpha Numeric Evaluation (SANE) score and Lysholm score above 75 points.[26] When these criteria are satisfied, our experience shows that the athlete is ready to initiate dynamic movements, attenuate ground force reaction forces, and provide the dynamic stability

---

Box 1
Baseline rehabilitation criteria for initiating return-to-sport phase

Subjective Knee Evaluation

Lysholm Score >75

SANE score >75

Normal performance of activities of daily living

Objective Knee Exam

No effusion

Full range of motion

Quadriceps muscle atrophy <2 cm

Strength Parameters

Single-leg press >70% of normal

Knee extension and flexion >70% of normal

Single-leg squat >60°

---

necessary to protect the repaired meniscus while progressively increasing the forces placed on the knee.

STATIC PHASE

The early phase of returning to sport focuses on core stabilization, return of single-leg strength, and reestablishing aerobic fitness. Static phase strength and balance training advances occur along a continuum as exercise progresses with the adherence to fundamental principles (**Box 2**). This spectrum begins with basic exercise and moves from slow, known, stable, low-force activities to fast, unknown, unstable, and high-force maneuvers that progressively recreate the stresses that are placed on the knee during athletic performance. These principles of progression are the core guidance that we use to return our athletes to sport.

The effects of weak core postural stabilizing muscle groups are magnified in the extremities and may place the knee in suboptimal biomechanical positions. Core strengthening develops a strong, stable axial musculoskeletal platform that is fundamental to the proper transfer of power to the extremities during sport. Initially bridging is emphasized, with concentration on proper technique (see **Fig. 1**). Once the athlete is able to confidently maintain this stable position, the trainer progresses them to less stable positions such as single-leg bridging or a placing the single leg on a ball

---

Box 2
Return-to-sport rehabilitation progression principles

- Low to high loads
- Slow to fast motions
- Stable to unstable platforms
- Uniplanar to multiplanar motions
- Concentrating to distracted performances

---

or foam pad. The stepwise progression of increased dynamic balancing activities challenges the athlete and assists in fine-tuning core stabilization.

Aerobic fitness should never be the limiting factor in the return-to-sport phase of training and with an in-season athlete this is rarely the case. However, for the more chronically injured athlete or one who has been unable to return to activities due to other injuries, particular emphasis should be placed on achieving a strong baseline cardiovascular fitness. This can be supplemented and maintained with early pool training, cycling, and finally with running on a treadmill. It is important to emphasize proper form in each of these activities to prevent breakdown in the kinetic chain, especially with treadmill running.

Continued training of the nonoperative leg during the period of injury and postoperative rehabilitation is critical because this leg may diminished strength and is essential as a control for the rehabilitation of the injured leg. Initiation of the return to sport phase for the noninjured leg is roughly 2 weeks before the operative knee is ready to begin. This helps return the uninjured leg return to full strength and also familiarizes the patient with the program they will use for the operative knee.

The single-leg squat and lunge are simple strengthening activities that are essential during this phase of return to sport after meniscal repair (**Fig. 2**). Despite an athlete's prior familiarity with these activities, breakdowns in form are common and often unrecognized by the patient. Supervision in the early phase is important to ensure proper technique, with vigilance as fatigue increases. It is not uncommon for an athlete to initially complain of subjective feelings of instability beyond 30° of flexion. Attaining the goal of 60° of flexion and the ability to hold the flexed position without quivering for 5 seconds before extending is an indication of progress in return of quadriceps muscle strength and control (**Fig. 3**).

As the athlete becomes proficient in the fundamental techniques, variations are added to restore balance and endurance that will be essential to the later functional application. The use of distraction techniques, such as catching a ball while performing single-leg squats or lunges, continue to challenge the athlete and reincorporate the normal proprioceptive stabilizing forces from the deliberate into the subconscious realm. Alterations in the position and incline of the support leg forces greater motor recruitment from the rehabilitating leg. Extending the number of repetitions and duration of the workout builds endurance. The rehab specialist must continue to closely observe the athlete with each new variation so that breakdowns in form are corrected and not incorporated as poor postural habits. The athlete has attained the key goals of this phase when they are strong, well balanced, and confident while performing these maneuvers.

DYNAMIC PHASE

Once the patient achieves static strength, he or she is ready to progress to more complex dynamic challenges that will advance the forces and demands to prepare for the on-field requirements placed on the rehabilitated knee. New to this phase are jumping and landing maneuvers, which place complex demands on the athlete. Exercises begin on 2 feet and in a single plane and progress to single-leg uniplanar vertical jump, single planar horizontal jumps, and eventually multilane jumps and landings from small heights. The rehabilitation specialist pays particular attention to landing with too little knee flexion or off balance.

As the athlete becomes proficient with each new set of maneuvers, new high-speed polymeric activities are introduced and timed for objective assessment of performance. The incorporation of single-leg hurdles (**Fig. 4**), box jumps, and zigzag

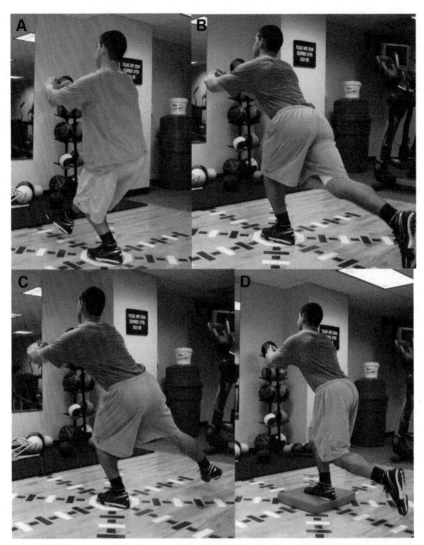

Fig. 2. Single-leg squat: This is an essential exercise during rehabilitation from meniscal repair. In addition to building strength, stability, and balance, it allows an accurate assessment of the strength of a single leg, without influence or compensation from the contralateral leg. Variations in supported leg position *(A)* forward, *(B)* backward, *(C)* to the side, and *(D)* standing on a foam pad force greater muscle recruitment and continue to challenge the athlete.

jumps develops multilane control. Dynamic maneuvers challenge the athlete both eccentrically and concentrically in a way that continues to recreate the unpredictable and varied environment in which the repaired meniscus and rehabilitated knee will be required to perform. Testing introduces a performance aspect that is familiar to the athlete and continues to advance the patient from deliberate, controlled actions to more natural motions and subconscious reactions. Essentially, the testing constitutes another form of distraction that forces the athlete to take his or her focus off of the

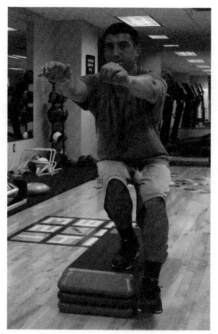

Fig. 3. Single-leg squat. When performed on a raised platform, the proficient athlete should be able to hold the flexed position for 5 seconds before extending. Varying the position of the supported leg will increase recruitment of core stabilizing muscles.

artificial controls of rehabilitation. If an athlete does not transition well in this phase, the rehabilitation specialist will continue to emphasize the fundamentals and can justify further restraint of the return to sport, even with an athlete eager to return to performance. Most athletes thrive on the introduction of performance goals, especially with the established confidence from the earlier phases of rehabilitation. The athlete is ready for progression when there is single-leg normalization within 15% of the uninjured side and consistent demonstration of good body mechanics, speed, and confidence.

BALLISTIC PHASE

By this point in the process, the athlete is relatively confident in his or her ability to return to sport, having mastered static and dynamic testing as well as the mechanics of jumping, landing, and change of direction. Ballistic progression emphasizes sport-specific high-load and high-speed maneuvers that simulate the on-field requirements of competition in a controlled environment. This phase relies heavily on the involvement and direction of an athletic trainer who is familiar with specific practice drills and can take the returning athlete through these drills in a protected setting.

Each sport and each position will place unique demands on the athlete, and during this phase, the athlete develops and demonstrates the ability to perform these activities. For basketball, this may be rebounding from the squatted position, pivoting while driving with the basketball or defensive slide drills. For the offensive linesman returning to football this may include firing out of a 3-point stance, while a cornerback must be able to change direction from a backpedal to a break on the ball at full speed.

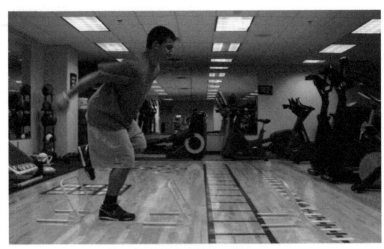

Fig. 4. Single leg hurdle. This is a more complex activity that the athlete progresses to after mastering the more fundamental maneuvers. Adding a timed performance component may be helpful.

The value of a close working relationship with a vigilant certified athletic trainer cannot be overemphasized. Observation of subtle signs of breakdown in core kinetics such as decreased knee flexion, poor postural control, or "leading" with the opposite leg must be recognized and addressed during this protected period before the athlete is released to return to full competition.

RETURN TO PLAY

In an ideal setting, athletes have their rehabilitation directed by a certified athletic trainer, or other similarly qualified professional, who is assigned to a specific sport and has daily communication with the coaching staff. This trainer attends practices and can supervise the returning athlete through return to unrestricted competition. By this point in the progression, there is a strong working relationship between the certified athletic trainer and the athlete which facilitates the detection of subtle weakness, confidence issues, and compensations. The final phase is return to

---

Box 3
Key points

1. Return to sport after meniscal repair is a process which comprehensively prepares the athlete for return to the playing field and may play as much or more of a role in a successful outcome as the surgical intervention itself.

2. There is a trend toward accelerated rehabilitation protocols after meniscal repair, which are supported by limited short-term data.

3. Returning an athlete to sport after meniscal repair is a multifactorial endeavor that must be individualized to the injury, biology, demands, and goals of the athlete.

4. To effectively guide an athlete from injury to return to competition, the involved physicians, physical therapist, athletic trainers, and coaches must work together as a team.

"limited" practice with "red jersey" or other similar designation. We have a policy with the coaching staff that these athletes are still under the authority of the certified athletic trainer, who has control of the intensity and duration of drills. In football, for example, the red jersey may return to noncontact portions of practice. This allows the certified athletic trainer to observe the athlete in a competitive environment against an opponent. As the athlete shifts the focus toward on-field performance, any compensation is difficult to hide. When the athlete performs well with one level of drills, the certified athletic trainer allows increased activity and eventually releases the athlete to full-speed competitive drills. The end result is an athlete ready for full return to competition with the confidence that every step was taken to restore the functioning meniscus and comprehensively prepare the athlete to return to sport (**Box 3**).

REFERENCES

1. Fairbank TJ. Knee joint changes after meniscectomy. J Bone Joint Surg Br 1948; 30B(4):664–70.
2. Shelbourne KD, Patel DV, Adsit WS, et al. Rehabilitation after meniscal repair. Clin Sports Med 1996;15(3):595–612.
3. Mintzer CM, Richmond JC, Taylor J. Meniscal repair in the young athlete. Am J Sports Med 1998;26(5):630–3.
4. Rosenberg TD, Scott SM, Coward DB, et al. Arthroscopic meniscal repair evaluated with repeat arthroscopy. Arthroscopy 1986;2(1):14–20.
5. Mooney M, Rosenberg TD. Meniscus repair: zone-specific technique. Sports Med Arthrosc Rev 1993;1:136–44.
6. Zhang ZN, Xu YK, Zhang WM, et al. Suture and immobilization of acute peripheral injuries of the meniscus in rabbits. Arthroscopy 1986;2(4):227–33.
7. Newman AP, Anderson DR, Daniels AU, et al. Mechanics of the healed meniscus in a canine model. Am J Sports Med 1989;17(2):164–75.
8. Dowdy PA, Miniaci A, Arnoczky SP, et al. The effect of cast immobilization on meniscal healing. An experimental study in the dog. Am J Sports Med 1995;23(6):721–8.
9. Salter RB, Simmonds DF, Malcolm BW, et al. The biological effect of continuous passive motion on the healing of full-thickness defects in articular cartilage. An experimental investigation in the rabbit. J Bone Joint Surg Am 1980;62(8):1232–51.
10. Eriksson E, Haggmark T. Comparison of isometric muscle training and electrical stimulation supplementing isometric muscle training in the recovery after major knee ligament surgery. A preliminary report. Am J Sports Med 1979;7(3):169–71.
11. DeHaven KE, Black KP, Griffiths HJ. Open meniscus repair. Technique and two to nine year results. Am J Sports Med 1989;17(6):788–95.
12. Fowler P, Pompan D. Rehabilitation after meniscal repair. Techniq Orthop 1993;8: 37–9.
13. Pyne SW. Current progress in meniscal repair and postoperative rehabilitation. Curr Sports Med Rep 2002;1(5):265–71.
14. Bowen TR, Feldmann DD, Miller MD. Return to play following surgical treatment of meniscal and chondral injuries to the knee. Clin Sports Med 2004;23(3):381–93, viii–ix.
15. Barber FA. Accelerated rehabilitation for meniscus repairs. Arthroscopy 1994;10(2): 206–10.
16. Bray RC, Smith JA, Eng MK, et al. Vascular response of the meniscus to injury: effects of immobilization. J Orthop Res 2001;19(3):384–90.
17. Richards DP, Barber FA, Herbert MA. Compressive loads in longitudinal lateral meniscus tears: a biomechanical study in porcine knees. Arthroscopy 2005;21(12): 1452–6.

18. Becker R, Wirz D, Wolf C, et al. Measurement of meniscofemoral contact pressure after repair of bucket-handle tears with biodegradable implants. Arch Orthop Trauma Surg 2005;125(4):254–60.
19. Starke C, Kopf S, Petersen W, et al. Meniscal repair. Arthroscopy 2009;25(9): 1033–44.
20. Brindle T, Nyland J, Johnson DL. The meniscus: review of basic principles with application to surgery and rehabilitation. J Athl Train 2001;36(2):160–9.
21. Mariani PP, Santori N, Adriani E, et al. Accelerated rehabilitation after arthroscopic meniscal repair: a clinical and magnetic resonance imaging evaluation. Arthroscopy 1996;12(6):680–6.
22. Jokl P, Stull PA, Lynch JK, et al. Independent home versus supervised rehabilitation following arthroscopic knee surgery–a prospective randomized trial. Arthroscopy 1989;5(4):298–305.
23. Moffet H, Richards CL, Malouin F, et al. Early and intensive physiotherapy accelerates recovery postarthroscopic meniscectomy: results of a randomized controlled study. Arch Phys Med Rehabil 1994;75(4):415–26.
24. Matthews P, St-Pierre DM. Recovery of muscle strength following arthroscopic meniscectomy. J Orthop Sports Phys Ther 1996;23(1):18–26.
25. Myer GD, Paterno MV, Ford KR, et al. Rehabilitation after anterior cruciate ligament reconstruction: criteria-based progression through the return-to-sport phase. J Orthop Sports Phys Ther 2006;36(6):385–402.
26. Lysholm J, Gillquist J. Evaluation of knee ligament surgery results with special emphasis on use of a scoring scale. Am J Sports Med 1982;10(3):150–4.

Partial Meniscus Substitution with Tissue-Engineered Scaffold: An Overview

Georgios Mouzopoulos, MD, MSc, Rainer Siebold, MD, Priv-Doz*

KEYWORDS

• Meniscal defect • Partial meniscal substitution
• Meniscal scaffold • Collagen meniscus implant
• Polyurethane meniscus implant

The fibrocartilaginous menisci and their insertions into bone represent a functional unit that plays an important role in the complex biomechanics of the knee joint.[1,2] Thanks to their firm attachement into bone, the menisci are able to reduce stress on the tibia, a function that is considered essential for articular cartilage protection and prevention of knee osteoarthritis.[3]

The concave shape of the superior surface and the flat inferior surface of the menisci, enhance the congruency between the femur and tibia.[4] The circumferential arrangement of type I collagen fibers provides the menisci with tensile strength, transmitting more than 50% of body weight in extension, and even more in flexion.[5] These structural properties allow the meniscus to perform many functions, such as distribution of stresses over the articular cartilage, absorption of shocks during axial loading, stabilization of the joint in both flexion and extension, and joint lubrication.[6,7] They also make a minor contribution toward secondary stabilization of the knee after cruciate ligament injuries.[8]

So, surgical removal of the meniscus can result in knee dysfunction and ultimately in secondary osteoarthritis because of increased peak stresses on the articular cartilage caused by a decreased contact area in the meniscectomized compartment.[9] Typically, the postmeniscectomy patients present with subtle joint line activity–related pain, induced by changes in the ambient barometric pressure and knee swelling.[10] Occasionaly, these patients might experience painful giving-way and crepitus.[11]

The authors have nothing to disclose.
Center for Knee & Foot Surgery, Sports Traumatology, ATOS Clinic Heidelberg, Bismarckstr. 9-15, 69115 Heidelberg, Germany
* Corresponding author.
E-mail address: rainer.siebold@atos.de

Clin Sports Med 31 (2012) 167–181
doi:10.1016/j.csm.2011.09.004
0278-5919/12/$ – see front matter © 2012 Elsevier Inc. All rights reserved.

Therefore, meniscal tissue should be preserved whenever possible.[12] However, in case of meniscectomy, replacement of the meniscus is supposed to decrease contact pressure on the articular cartilage surface. So it seems to be a logical approach to improve function, relieve pain, and prevent further articular cartilage degeneration.[2,4,6,10,11]

Although allograft meniscal transplantation is a viable option in selected knees, there are substantial issues related to the availability, preservation techniques, the individual shaping of the meniscus and complications such as delayed or incomplete biologic incorporation, the potential for an immune response that will hinder graft healing, and the risk of disease transmission.[10,11] Taking into consideration all these limitations, tissue-engineering approaches hold tremendous promise for biologic substitution of meniscal tissue by a meniscal shaped scaffold.

This article focuses on partial meniscus substitution with tissue-engineered scaffolds for the treatment of symptomatic meniscal defects after partial meniscectomy.

TYPES OF TISSUE-ENGINEERED MENISCAL SCAFFOLDS

Currently, there are 2 tissue-engineered scaffolds in clinical use: a collagen meniscal scaffold (Menaflex, ReGen Biologics Inc) and a polyurethane meniscal scaffold (Actifit, Orteq Bioengineering, Ltd). Both are biodegradable implants and have been suggested as a matrix to enable the body's own tissue to fill the segmental loss after partial meniscectomy.[2,13] Menaflex (formerly CMI) collagen meniscus scaffold was cleared for sale in Europe and other countries in 2000 for the replacement of medial meniscus and in 2006 for the replacement of lateral meniscus.[1] The name *CMI* was used for the Menaflex during the early phase of the implant. The Actifit received the CE Mark in July 2008 for the replacement either medial or lateral meniscus.[14]

MECHANICAL AND BIOLOGIC PROPERTIES

The Menaflex (ReGen Biologics Inc) is a degradable and biocompatible scaffold composed of purified type I collagen fabricated from bovine Achilles tendon.[11] The tendon tissue is trimmed and minced, and the type I collagen fibers are purified by using various chemical treatments, such as enzymes to remove noncollagenous materials and lipids.[10] A mixture made up of hyalouronic acid and chondroitin sulphate is added and the product is homogenized and enriched with glycosamino-glycans to allow cellular ingrowth. Finally, the fibers are moulded and cross-linked then sterilized to make meniscus-shaped tissue. The collagen meniscus implant has been tested extensively in vitro and in laboratory animal trials.[15–18] Many studies have already reported that the collagen scaffold could support ingrowth and maturation of meniscus fibrochondrocytes and the development of a mature and functional new tissue matrix.[15–18] In the porcine animal model, the implant was rapidly reabsorbed in 1 to 2 years, but human data suggest that the implant is absorbed more slowly.[10]

The Actifit (Orteq Bioengineering Ltd) is a highly interconnected porous polymeric flexible and degradable scaffold, which provides support while allowing the ingrowth of new tissue.[14] This polyurethane implant is a honeycomblike structure consisting of 2 domains, a polyester soft segment (80%) and an aliphatic polyurethane hard segment.[19] The soft segment is a biodegradable polyester that allows the transformation into meniscuslike tissue, as the material slowly degrades over time. Histologic biopsies of the regenerated tissue in dogs showed fibrous connective tissue that is differentiating toward fibrochondrocytic matrix.[20] These biopsy findings show that host cells (most likely derived from synovium or synovial fluid) can migrate into the meniscus implant material, differentiate into fibrochondrocytelike cells containing proteoglycans and type II collagen, and synthesize appropriate matrix molecules.[20]

Box 1
Indications and contraindications for tissue-engineered meniscal scaffolds[2,4]

Indications

History of partial meniscectomy

Pain and/or swelling caused by partial meniscectomy

Failed conservative treatment

Willingness to follow slow rehabilitation

Contraindications

Total meniscectomy

Advanced arthritis (late grade III or IV)

Flattening of the femoral condyle

Marked osteophyte formation

Inflammatory arthritis

Synovial disease

History of knee infections

Immunodeficiency

Obesity (body mass index >35)

Systemic metabolic diseases

Skeletal immaturity

Relative contraindications

Ligamentous instability

Malalignment

The synthetic implant material is resorbed gradually and replaced by this newly formed tissue.[19] The degradation mechanism takes place in the presence of water through hydrolysis.[14] Three months after implantation, complete infiltration of all pores of the implant with vascularized fibrous tissue is evidenced, and 3 months later the scaffold is integrated with the peripheral capsule and is completely filled with tissue.[13] Usually after 1.5 years the molecular weight of the polyourethane decreases to 50% of its molecular weight, and the degradation process is completed after 4 to 6 years.[14] The hard segment is semidegradable and acts as filler and multifunctional crosslink and is very important for the mechanical strength of the material.[19]

Both Menaflex and Actifit are available in 2 configurations, shaped like a medial and lateral meniscus, to fit the corresponding meniscal defect.[3,14]

INDICATIONS AND CONTRAINDICATIONS

The indications and contraindications for a partial meniscal substitution are listed in **Box 1**. The ideal candidate for a partial meniscal substitution is young complains of moderate-to-severe pain after partial meniscetomy, is not significantly overweight (body mass index <35), has a well-aligned stable knee and should rather have a focal cartilage damage according to the International Cartilage Repair Society.[10,14]

Partial meniscal substitution may also be indicated for acute partial meniscectomies not yet affected by chronic (painful) disability.[14] And although it may yield superior clinical results, prophylactic implantation of a meniscal scaffold without symptoms after meniscectomy is not recommended to date.[21]

An important technical aspect for the implantation of a meniscal scaffold is an intact meniscal rim and popliteal bridge to enable attachment of implant and cellular ingrowth.[14] In case of subtotal meniscectomy, with nearly all of the native meniscus destroyed or removed, the use of a human meniscal allograft may be indicated.[10]

Comorbitities, such as ligamentous instability, malalignment, and cartilage degeneration are considered relative contraindications and should be addressed before or at the time of partial meniscus subtitution.[2,11] Patients with focal chondral defects of the condyles or an ACL deficiency are considered candidates for scaffold implantation as long as these lesions are appropriately corrected. Similarly, when patients have had secondary varus or valgus deformities caused by a meniscectomy in the past, this deformity has to be corrected simultaneously or in a staged fashion.[9]

SURGICAL TECHNIQUE

The procedure is performed arthroscopically and requires standard anteromedial and anterolateral portals.[9,10,14] The damaged portion of the meniscus is resected, and the defect is extended into the vascularized red-red zone, leaving a stable and potentially bleeding rim, ensuring smooth margins of the debrided defect.[10,14] The remnants of the native tissue are left intact.[2,10] The meniscal rim is punctured to create potential vascular access channels to enhance healing.[14] Also, gentle rasping of the synovial lining is performed to stimulate bleeding and better incorporation of the meniscal scaffold.

The length of the meniscal defect is measured with an arthroscopic ruler (**Fig. 1**). The meniscal scaffold is then cut accordingly.[9–11] To ensure an optimal fit into the

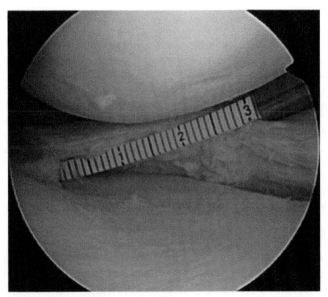

Fig. 1. Arthroscopic measurement of defect size in posterior horn of medial meniscus with spezial ruler.

prepared meniscal defect, it is recommended to oversize the meniscal scaffold by 3 mm for defects less than 3 cm and by 5 mm for defects greater than 3 cm.[14] It is very important to be precise with measuring and cutting of the scaffold to avoid an intra-articular mismatch. After marking of the surface for better orientation, the implant is then delivered through an enlarged arthroscopic portal in the joint and is positioned into the meniscal defect.

Fixation to the native meniscus rim may be performed with nonabsorbable sutures (size 2.0, polyester or polypropylene and braided or monofil sutures) using an inside-out or outside-in technique.[3,9] Alternatively, an all-inside technique with all-inside implants may be used. The type of suturing depends on the preference of the surgeon as well as the location of the defect. Generally, horizontal mattress sutures are used in the anterior (outside-in technique) and posterior (all-inside technique) margins, and vertical mattress sutures (a minimum of 5 mm apart for medial meniscus and 10 mm apart for lateral meniscus) placed at one-third to one-half of the implants height are used along the body rim.[3,9,14] An arthroscopic example after implantation of an Actifit scaffold into a symptomatic posterior horn defect of the medial meniscus is shown in **Fig. 2**.

POSTOPERATIVE REHABILITATION

The patients should understand and strictly follow the specific rehabilitation program to enhance implant healing and to protect the newly formed meniscuslike tissue from potentially harmful stresses. **Table 1** presents the recommended postoperative rehabilitation protocol for meniscal scaffolds.[10,14]

CLINICAL OUTCOMES

The clinical outcomes after Menaflex are presented in **Table 2**. Clinical studies suggest that the collagen implant Menaflex can safely replace the tissue after partial

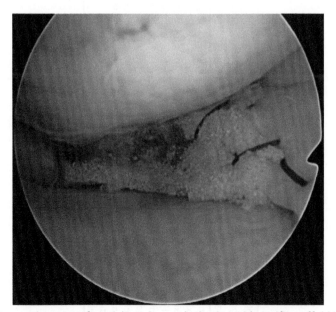

Fig. 2. Arthroscopic aspect of partial meniscus substitution with Actifit scaffold in posterior horn defect of medial meniscus.

Table 1
Rehabilitation program recommended after synthetic graft transplantation[10,14]

1st–3rd Wk	4th–6th Wk	9th–13th Wk	14th–20th Wk	6th Month	9th Month
Non weight bearing	Partial weight bearing increasing gradually	Full weight bearing with brace	Full weight bearing without brace	Hydrotherapy	Participating in contact sports
Flexion to 30° (1st–2nd wk)	Flexion to 90° (4th–5th wk)	Closed chain hamstrings exercise	Increased open and closed chain lower extremity exercises	Swimming (crawl, breaststroke)	
Flexion to 60° (3rd wk)	Partial wall sits under 90° (5th wk)	Lunges between 0 and 90°	Jogging on level ground	Participating in contact sports	
Full extension	Full flexion (6th wk)	Proprioception exercises	Plyometrics		
Isometric quadriceps exercises		Dynamic quadriceps exercises	Sport-related exercises without pivoting		
Patella mobilization					
Heel slides					
Quad sets					
Anti-equinous foot exercises					
Achilles tendon stretching					

meniscectomy.[2,3,9–11,22] All of the biopsy studies showed infiltration of the implant by cells similar to fibroblasts as well as the development of a blood supply, which enhances new cell growth.[2,9,10,15] The implant seems to be well tolerated because there is no evidence of an inflammatory infiltrate on histology examinations.[2,9] The average pain scores decreased significantly, and knee function, measured by the Lysholm scale, as well as patients' activity levels increased.[2,3,9,10,15] In a study by Bulgheroni and colleagues[10] of 34 patients, no development of osteoarthritis was seen after 5 years of follow-up on x-rays The conclusion of the aforementioned study was that the presence of the collagen meniscus scaffold did remain in place for more than 5 years without causing any negative effects in the knee joint.[9,10] It allowed returning to physical activity and showed histologic characteristics of meniscuslike tissue.[2,10,15] This supported the concept that a collagen meniscus scaffold can be used to replace irreparable or removed meniscus tissue.[1,2]

Unfortunately, there was no description of the integrity of the Menaflex scaffold at the time of second-look arthroscopies. Moreover, without controls, it is unclear whether the symptomatic improvements are owing to the meniscal scaffold or the partial meniscectomy. Therefore, Rodkey and coworkers[9] performed a randomized, multicenter study to prove the superiority of the implantation of a collagen scaffold over a partial meniscectomy performed alone.[9] The trial was designed with 2 concurrent study arms. One arm of the trial included patients with no previous surgery on the involved meniscus (designated as the "acute" arm of the study), and the second arm included patients who had experienced one or more surgical procedures on the involved meniscus (designated as the "chronic" arm). Patients participating in the study were randomly assigned either to receive the collagen meniscus implant or to serve as controls receiving only partial meniscectomy without implantation. In the acute group, 75 patients received a collagen meniscus implant and 82 were controls. In the chronic group, 85 patients received the implant and 69 were controls. The mean duration of follow-up was 59 months (range, 16 to 92 months). The 141 repeat arthroscopies done at 1 year showed that the collagen meniscus implants had resulted in significantly ($P = .001$) increased meniscal tissue compared with that seen after the original index partial meniscectomy. The implant supported meniscuslike matrix production and integration as it was assimilated and resorbed. In the chronic group, the patients who had received an implant regained significantly more of their lost activity than did the controls ($P = .02$) and they underwent significantly fewer nonprotocol reoperations ($P = .04$). No differences were detected between the 2 treatment groups in the acute arm of the study. The authors concluded that the collagen meniscus implant has the utility to be used to replace irreparable or lost meniscal tissue in patients with a chronic meniscal injury. However, the implant was not found to have any benefit for patients with an acute injury.

Zaffagnini and colleagues[23] reported on 17 patients with partial meniscectomy plus collagen meniscus transplantation for irreparable meniscus lesion and 16 patients with partial meniscectomy alone. After 11 years of follow-up, the authors reported significantly lower pain, higher scores according to the International Knee Documentation Committee (IKDC) and Tegner less medial joint space narrowing in patients treated with collagen meniscus implantation. Although these results seem to be promising, it should be mentioned that patients' assignments to each type of treatment was not random, and the choice was made by the patients themselves. In fact, the older patients decided to receive only partial meniscectomy. So it remains unclear whether the clinical improvement is due to the partial meniscectomy performed alone or the collagen scaffold.

Table 2
Studies reporting clinical outcomes after collagen meniscal implantation (Menaflex)

Author	Study	Patients (follow-up)	Clinical Findings	Second-Look Arthroscopy	X-Ray/MRI Findings	Histology Findings	Conclusion
Stone et al[11] (1997)	—	9 (3 y)	30% reduction in pain (VAS scale) Improvement in Tegner score 22% reoperation rate	Performed only in 1 case and showed new tissue replacing the implant	On X-ray no medial compartment degeneration	New tissue similar to native meniscus	Regeneration of meniscal cartilage through a collagen scaffold is possible
Steadman et al[2] (2005)	Prospective	8 (5.8 y)	No symptoms in all patients Improvement in Lysholm score from 75 to 88 points and in Tegner score from 3 to 6 No complications	The newly grown tissue appeared grossly meniscuslike The tissue was indistinguishable from native meniscus Average 69% of the defects were filled	On X-ray no medial compartment degeneration On MRI no or little change of chondral surfaces and signal almost similar to mature fibrocartilage of native meniscus	The cells had the appearance of normal meniscus fibrochondrocytes and no inflammatory infiltrates were observed	The meniscuslike tissue that developed after collagen meniscus implant placement maintained its structure and function

Linke et al[1] (2006)	Prospective, randomized	23 (2 y)	—	In these patients the authors performed high tibial osteotomy and collagen meniscus implantation. > 50% reduction in pain (VAS scale) Improvement in Lysholm score from 65 to 90 points and in IKDC score from 60 to 83	Performed in 23 patients after 8–12 months follow up revealed: 34.7% of cases complete healing 30.4% of cases partial healing 34.9% of cases no healing with only small remnants of the implant left	—	The efficacy of meniscus implantation is not clear because there is no significant difference in outcomes after high tibia osteotomy performed alone or after combined high tibia osteotomy and meniscus collagen implantation
Genovese et al[22] (2007)	—	40 (2 y)	—	30% reoperation rate	On MRI 5% of cases with new chondral lesions Interface between implant and native meniscus in 17.5% of cases Signal similar to native meniscus only in 25%	—	The MRI signal of the implant is different from the natural structure

(continued on next page)

Table 2
(continued)

Author	Study	Patients (follow-up)	Clinical findings	Second-look arthroscopy	X-ray/MRI findings	Histology findings	Conclusion
Zaffagnini et al[3] (2007)	Prospective	8 (6.8 y)	Absence of pain in 50% of patients Range of motion compared with opposite leg was normal in 62.5% of patients IKDC score evaluation showed improvement in 75% of patients no complications	Revealed intact chondral surface and the presence of the implant tissue in 2 out of 3 cases at 2 years follow up The size of the implant was reduced in 2 cases and disappeared in 1 case at 2 years follow-up	On X-ray no medial compartment degeneration in 75% of patients MRI evaluation showed mixoid degeneration signal at the implant site in 62.5% of cases	—	The implant could reduce the deterioration of the knee joint despite of its abnormal aspect

| Rodkey et al[9] (2008) | Prospective | 160 (5 y) | Improvement in Lysholm score, average 21 points
The patients regained the 42% of their lost activity level
Probably or at least possibly related to the collagen meniscus implant in 4.3% of patients
9.5% reoperation rate | Grossly meniscuslike new tissue was observed after 1 year follow-up
No chondral damage caused by implant or new tissue was observed after 1 year follow-up
Average 70.5% filling of the defect | Demonstrated some degree of assimilation of the collagen meniscus implant into a newly developing fibrochondrocytic matrix in all patients
Inflammation of the synovium observed in <5% of the cases | Safe implant adequate to enhance knee function especially in chronic injuries |
| Bulgheroni et al[10] (2010) | Prospective | 34 (5 y) | Improvement in Lysholm score, average 36 points and improvement in Tegner score from 2 to 5 at 2 years' follow-up
21% reoperation rate | The implant not completely reabsorbed at 5 years
Only slight reduction of the implant in most cases | On X-ray no progression of osteoarthritis
On MRI signal not similar to native meniscus, no further chondral degeneration | Tissue not completely similar to normal meniscus | No negative effects of the implant |

(continued on next page)

Table 2
(continued)

Author	Study	Patients (follow-up)	Clinical findings	Second-look arthroscopy	X-ray/MRI findings	Histology findings	Conclusion
Zaffagnini et al[23] (2011)	Prospective	17 (11.08 y)	83% reduction of pain (VAS scale) High IKDC and Tegner scores Almost 50% improvent in Lysholm score Improvement in SF-36 score 23.5% reoperation rate	-	On X-ray no progression of osteoarthritis On MRI 4 (23.5%) patients with normal signal, 11 (64.7%) patients with myxoid degeneration signal, 2 (11.7%) patients with no recognizable implant		Clinical and radiologic outcomes significantly improved even after long-term periods

In cases of subtotal medial meniscectomy associated with varus knee, several authors recommend to perform a high tibial osteotomy (HTO) in combination with a collagen meniscus implantation.[3,9,10] However, Linke and coworkers[1] in a randomized, prospective study, treated 23 patients with HTO and collagen meniscus implantation and 16 patients with HTO performed alone. After 2 years of follow-up, the authors reported no significant differences between the 2 groups regarding the Lysholm and IKDC scores. Unfortunately, the authors did not mention if significant differences were existing in the preoperative setting regarding these scores. From their scores, one may conclude that patients who were treated with HTO alone deteriorated over time in terms of knee functionality in contrast to patients who received combined treatment. Interestingly, during second-look arthroscopy 8 to 12 months after implantation, the authors found 34.7% of cases with complete healing of the implant, 30.4% of partial healing, and 34.9% without healing and only small remnants of the implant left.

Since the Actifit implant received the approval for the treatment of medial or lateral irreparable partial meniscal tears recently in July 2008, there are no long-term studies reporting clinical results after implanting this scaffold. The only clinical study existing in the literature is reported by Verdonk and coworkers.[13] They reported 1-year results of a clinical multicenter study including 9 centers throughout Europe. Fifty-two patients (34 medial and 18 lateral) were treated with an Actifit implantation.[13] According to the observations of the 10 surgeons who participated in the study as investigators, at 3 months after implantation, the Dynamic Contrast-Enhanced Magnet Resonance Imaging showed evidence of tissue ingrowth into the peripheral half of the scaffold in 81.4% of patients. Also, biopsy samples obtained by second-look arthroscopy 1 year after implantation showed fully vital material, with no signs of necrosis or cell death, without serious adverse reaction to the scaffold material or its degradation products. At the same time during second-look arthroscopy, integration of the scaffold with the native meniscus was observed in 97.7% of patients. Magnetic resonance imaging (MRI) scans showed stable articular cartilage grades in the index compartment between the 1-week and the 12-month follow-up in 88.6% of patients. The authors concluded that using the acellular polyurethane scaffold to treat irreparable partial meniscus tissue lesions is a a reliable and safe option. Surely, long-term studies are needed to obtain based evidence results. Unfortunately, there was no description of the integrity of the Actifit scaffold at the time of second-look arthroscopy. The 2-year results of above multicenter-study are accepted for publication in the American Journal of Sports Medicine. The authors report stable or improved International Cartilage Repair Society cartilage grades in 92.5% of subjects between baseline and 24 months. The incidence of treatment failure was 9 (17.3%) subjects: 3 (8.8%) in subjects with medial meniscus lesions and 6 (33.3%) in subjects with lateral meniscus lesions. Clinically and statistically significant improvements ($P<.0001$) compared with baseline were reported from 6 to 24 months in all clinical outcomes scores (visual analog scale, IKDC, Knee Injury and Osteoarthritis Outcome Score including Sport and Recreation subscale and Lysholm), showing improvements in both pain and function. The authors concluded that 2 years after implantation, safety and clinical outcome data from their study support the use of the polyurethane scaffold for the treatment of irreparable, painful, partial meniscus lesions.

No studies exist in the literature comparing the clinical outcome between patients who received a meniscal allograft or a meniscal scaffold for the treatment of meniscal defects. Van der Wal and colleagues[4] reported the outcomes for 63 meniscal allografts after a mean follow-up of 13.8 years. However, despite a significant improvement in function overall, there was a 29% long-term failure rate.[4] Stollsteimer and colleagues[24] stated that although patients continue to have good pain relief after their meniscal allograft transplantation, the average shrinkage in the size of the meniscus as shown on MRI is of concern.[24] As a matter of fact meniscus allografts are used to replace the entire meniscus; however, the meniscal scaffolds are designed to substitute only a partial meniscal defect, eg, posterior horn of lateral or medial meniscus.[2,9,10,14,25,26]

SUMMARY

The desired degradable bioengineered meniscal scaffold should provide a matrix framework for restoration of vascular, cell, and matrix elements of the tissue; should present high interconnectivity, allowing easy diffusion of nutrients and waste products; should contain a large pore volume (pore size between 150 and 500 μm) and high surface area; should provide the best ingrowth of mesenchymal tissue and the least inflammatory response; and should optimize the process of degradation in relation with tissue restoration.[27] Clinically, the implant should be chondroprotective, restore normal biomechanical meniscus kinematics within the joint, provide pain relief, and have no deleterious effects on surrounding tissue and should be able to integrate with the host tissue.[28]

Both bioengineered meniscal scaffolds do meet most of the properties of the desired scaffold and may, therefore, be recommended for the treatment of irreparable partial meniscus defects.[1-3,9,10] Although the above-mentioned studies showed successful meniscuslike tissue ingrowth into the scaffolds, the clinical mid- to long-term benefit of these implants is not yet clear. A point of concern of scaffolds is substance loss over time as well as breakage of the implant, which may lead to the unanswered question of long-term survivership and their biomechanical value.

Prospective, randomized studies with long-term follow-up are needed, comparing both meniscal scaffolds and control patients after partial meniscectomy to provide based evidence knowledge about the clinical efficacy. Also, long-term MRI studies could be helpful in determining the integrity of the scaffolds over the time.

REFERENCES

1. Linke R, Ulmer M, Imhoff A. Replacement of the meniscus with a collagen implant (CMI). Oper Orthop Traumatol 2006;18(5-6):453–62.
2. Steadman JR, Rodkey WG. Tissue-engineered collagen meniscus implants: 5- to 6-year feasibility study results. Arthroscopy 2005;21(5):515–25.
3. Zaffagnini S, Giordano G, Vascellari A, et al. Arthroscopic collagen meniscus implant results at 6 to 8 years follow up. Knee Surg Sports Traumatol Arthrosc 2007;15(2): 175–83.
4. van der Wal RJ, Thomassen BJ, van Arkel ER. Long-term clinical outcome of open meniscal allograft transplantation. Am J Sports Med 2009;37(11):2134–9.
5. Konan S, Rayan F, Haddad FS. Do physical diagnostic tests accurately detect meniscal tears? Knee Surg Sports Traumatol Arthrosc 2009;17(7):806–11.
6. Verdonk P, Demurie A, Almqvist K, et al. Transplantation of viable meniscal allograft. Survivorship analysis and clinical outcome of one hundred cases. J Bone Joint Surg Am 2005;87(4):715–24.
7. Verdonk P, Verstraete K, Almqvist K, et al. Meniscal allograft transplantation: long term clinical results with radiological and magnetic resonance imaging correlations. Knee Surg Sports Traumatol Arthrosc 2006;14:694–706.
8. Rayan F, Bhonsle S, Shukla DD. Clinical, MRI, and arthroscopic correlation in meniscal and anterior cruciate ligament injuries. Int Orthop 2009;33(1):129–32.

9. Rodkey WG, DeHaven KE, Montgomery WH III, et al. Comparison of the collagen meniscus implant with partial meniscectomy. A prospective randomized trial. J Bone Joint Surg Am 2008;90(7):1413–26.

10. Bulgheroni P, Murena L, Ratti C, et al. Follow-up of collagen meniscus implant patients: clinical, radiological, and magnetic resonance imaging results at 5 years. Knee 2010;17(3):224–9.

11. Stone KR, Steadman JR, Rodkey WG, et al. Regeneration of meniscal cartilage with use of a collagen scaffold. Analysis of preliminary data. J Bone Joint Surg Am 1997;79(12):1770–7.

12. Herrlin S, Hallander M, Wange P, et al. Arthroscopic or conservative treatment of degenerative medial meniscal tears: a prospective randomised trial. Knee Surg Sports Traumatol Arthrosc 2007;15(4):393–401.

13. Verdonk R, Verdonk P, Heinrichs E, et al. Tissue ingrowth after implantation of a novel, biodegradable polyurethane scaffold for treatment of partial meniscal lesions. Am J Sports Med 2011;39(4):774–82.

14. de Groot J. Actifit, polyurethane meniscus implant: basic science. In: Beaufils P, Verdonk R, editors. The meniscus. Heidelberg: Springer-Verlag; 2010. p. 383–7.

15. Stone KR, Rodkey WG, Webber RJ, et al. Meniscal regeneration with copolymeric collagen scaffolds: in vitro and in vivo studies evaluated clinically, histologically, biochemically. Am J Sports Med 1992;20:104–11.

16. Stone KR, Rodkey WG, Webber RJ, et al. Development of a prosthetic meniscal replacement. In: Mow VC, Arnoczky SP, Jackson DJ, editors. Knee meniscus: basic and clinical foundation. New York: Raven Press; 1992. p. 165–73.

17. Steadman JR, Rodkey WG, Li S-T. The collagen meniscus implant. Development and clinical trials of a device to treat meniscus injuries of the knee. Sports Orthop Traumatol 2000;16:173–7.

18. Rodkey WG, Stone KR, Steadman JR. Prosthetic meniscal replacement. In: Finerman GAM, Noyes FR, editors. Biology and biomechanics of the traumatized synovial joint: the knee as a model. Rosemont (IL): American Academy of Orthopaedic Surgeons; 1992. p. 222–31.

19. Verdonk R, Verdonk P, Heinrichs E. Polyurethane meniscus implant: technique. In: Beaufils P, Verdonk R, editors. The meniscus. Heidelberg: Springer-Verlag; 2010. p. 389–94.

20. Tienen TG, Heijkants RG, de Groot JH, et al. Replacement of the knee meniscus by a porous polymer implant: a study in dogs. Am J Sports Med 2006;34(1):64–71.

21. Verdonk R, Almqvist KF, Huysse W, et al. Meniscal allografts: indications and outcomes. Sports Med Arthrosc 2007;15(3):121–5.

22. Genovese E, Angeretti MG, Ronga M, et al. Follow-up of collagen meniscus implants by MRI. Radiol Med 2007;112(7):1036–48.

23. Zaffagnini S, Marcheggiani Muccioli GM, Lopomo N, et al. Prospective long-term outcomes of the medial collagen meniscus implant versus partial medial meniscectomy: a minimum 10-year follow-up study. Am J Sports Med 2011;39(5):977–85.

24. Stollsteimer GT, Shelton WR, Dukes A, et al. Meniscal allograft transplantation: a 1 to 5 year follow up of 22 patients. Arthroscopy 2000;16(4):343–7.

25. Wirth JC, Peters G, Milachowski KA, et al. Long-term results of meniscal allograft transplantation. Am J Sports Med 2002;30:174–81.

26. Rodeo SA. Meniscal allografts—where do we stand? Am J Sports Med 2001;29: 246–61.

27. Arnoczky SP. Building a meniscus. Biologic considerations. Clin Orthop 1999;367: S244–53.

28. Arnoczky SP. Meniscus. Clin Orthop 1999;367:S293–5.

Index

Note: Page numbers of article titles are in **boldface** type.

Clin Sports Med 31 (2012) 183–186
doi:10.1016/S0278-5919(11)00115-3
0278-5919/12/$ – see front matter © 2012 Elsevier Inc. All rights reserved.

sportsmed.theclinics.com

Printed and bound by CPI Group (UK) Ltd, Croydon, CR0 4YY

03/10/2024

01040446-0017